Matthew's Enigma

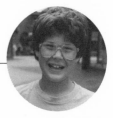

Matthew's Enigma

A Father's Portrait of His Autistic Son

Matei Calinescu

TRANSLATED BY
Angela Jianu

Indiana University Press
Bloomington · Indianapolis

This book is a publication of

Indiana University Press
601 North Morton Street
Bloomington, IN 47404-3797 USA

http://iupress.indiana.edu

Telephone orders 800-842-6796
Fax orders 812-855-7931
Orders by e-mail iuporder@indiana.edu

The paper used in this publication meets
the minimum requirements of American
National Standard for Information
Sciences—Permanence of Paper for Printed
Library Materials, ANSI Z39.48-1984.

Manufactured in the United States of America

Library of Congress Cataloging-in-Publication
Data

Calinescu, Matei.
  [Portretul lui M. English]
  Matthew's enigma : a father's portrait of his
autistic son / Matei Calinescu ; translated by
Angela Jianu.
    p. cm.
  Includes bibliographical references.
  ISBN 978-0-253-35297-2 (cloth : alk. paper)
  — ISBN 978-0-253-22066-0 (pbk. : alk.
paper) 1. Calinescu, Adrian M., 1977–2003.
2. Autistic children—Biography. 3. Autistic
children—Family relationships. 4. Autistic
youth—Biography. I. Title.
  RJ506.A9C3513 2009
  618.92'858820092—dc22
  [B]

                                    2008027739

1 2 3 4 5 14 13 12 11 10 09

Contents

Preface

This is a biographical portrait of my son, Matthew, who was born on 24 August 1977 in Bloomington, Indiana, and who died on 1 March 2003 in his hometown, not yet twenty-six. It was written during the forty days after his death, the forty symbolic days that follow all deaths. Throughout those days I was incapable of anything but thinking of him as I wrote, transcribing fragments from my intermittent diaries, trying to capture the fragile truth of memories which haunted me and which, I knew, would inevitably be lost in the dusk of time. I did not count the days, but it so happened that on the fortieth I felt reconciled to my pain, almost serene in my sadness. The outcome is this reflection on his life, and also on that part of my life when I did my best to understand the enigma he embodied. I never did, but I gained a different insight—that he was, in his own way and in the way he continues to live in my memory, a gift. God's gift? I cannot be sure, but his name, which is also mine, contains a divine echo of that gift from the depths of biblical etymology. A name is a sign, it has often been said—*nomen est omen*—but the omen is always indecipherable: it is a small mystery wrapped within a greater mystery, one that is in fact infinite.

I have written this book for myself as a kind of spiritual exercise, but I do hope it may help others. This is what prompts me to offer it for publication. I wish to thank my wife, Uca, and my daughter, Irena, for reading the manuscript, adding memories and making useful suggestions. The English edition of this book differs from the original Romanian edition of *Portretul lui M* (2003) in two ways: first, it is shorter (I decided to leave out a few chapters that were, I thought, of little interest to a non-Romanian reader); second, and more important, I changed the order of the chapters, particularly in the first half, to give the chronology of Matthew's story, as well as that of my discovery of his condition, a firmer and more dramatic outline. I owe the idea of this restructuring to Breon Mitchell, who read the manuscript of the English translation twice over, also making numerous suggestions for stylistic improvements. I have a great debt of gratitude to him. Many thanks are also due to Norman Manea, who read the original version of the book and made many insightful comments. Candace McNulty copyedited the manuscript with numerous useful suggestions, for which I am grateful. My heartfelt thanks also go to my friends and colleagues who read the current English version: Scott Russell Sanders, Alvin H. Rosenfeld, Stine Levy, and, last but not least, to Janet Rabinowitch for her generous editorial help.

Matthew's
Enigma

Chapter One

Pages from an Old Diary

❋ **26 AUGUST 1977**

Two days ago my son Matthew was born at Bloomington Hospital, at 6:29 AM. Weight: 8½ lb. I was there with Uca the whole time, holding her hand and trying to help with her labor pains by joining in the Lamaze breathing exercises we had trained for over the last three months.

❋ **27 AUGUST 1977**

Uca and Matthew leave hospital. Uca happy. Matthew is a child we wanted, loved and worshipped by his mother from the first. He is going to be happy.

❋ **4 JUNE 1978**

. . . Last week, on 27 May, all five of us (my mother was visiting and Irena was with us, of course) to Chicago, to have Matthew baptized in the Romanian church there—St. Mary's. Christinel and Mircea Eliade were his godparents. We only stayed in Chicago one day—we were back on the 28th—but it was truly enjoyable. Matthew was charming [. . .] the beauty of the naked child in the almost deserted church, the afternoon sunlight that filtered, golden-speckled, through the windows. Just that moment alone, in that beautiful light . . .

✳ 11 JUNE 1979

During a lengthy afternoon walk with Matthew in his carriage, I stopped at the Glass Harmonica, the only good classical music store in Bloomington, and bought Franck's Sonata for violin and piano (Heifetz/Rubinstein), also his Piano Quintet . . .

✳ 14 JUNE 1979

I notice in Matthew an interesting type of memory, extremely individualized, manifesting itself among other things by the high ratio of proper names he has memorized before the age of two. He knows all our neighbors' names and, of course, those of all the children on our street, whom he immediately recognizes at a distance. This way of grasping names (do other two-year-olds share it?) predisposes him to treat many common nouns as proper names. Birds, dogs, cats—the animals he is familiar with—he refers to as though they were persons. When they disappear from sight, he waves to them, saying: "Bye-bye, bird," "Bye-bye, doggie," "Bye-bye, cat," "Bye-bye, squirrel," in the same way that he addresses the blonde and very energetic little daughter of our neighbors, of whom he is very fond: "Bye-bye, Anna," with a beaming smile. Even more striking and amusing is his notion—amusing to him, as well—that, seen from a different angle, the same animal or object becomes a different animal or object. As Mrs. Farmer's black tomcat strolls back and forth in front of him, he exclaims at short intervals, surprised and cheerful: "Another cat!" "Another cat!" This reminds me of Borges's story "Funes, el memorioso," which, interpreted in this light, could be seen as a detailed analysis (with that strangely rigorous logic of Borges) of infantile perception, so sensitive to issues of identity that any change in space through movement appears as a change of identity and any repetition appears as pure novelty. Certainly, in Funes this childish trait—this quasi-Platonic quality of perception—was associated with hypermnesia: for Funes remembered every leaf of every tree he had seen, as well as every time he had seen it. He suffered from a condition from which, in a different way, Borges himself, with his prodigious memory, suffered—or benefited. But would it not be correct to say that this "auroral" perception is more natural, more in keeping with the essential nature of things? Immobility should be the ideal. In this light, movement—the lazy walk of Mrs. Farmer's tom—is an object of amazement.

✳ 5 JULY 1979

Long walk with Matthew in his carriage. He is exceptionally sweet, and becomes even sweeter when I buy him a lollipop from Booknook, where I also buy the *New York Times*. Then we stop at the Glass Harmonica, where I cannot resist the temptation of buying a piece by John Cage (for prepared piano) . . .

✳ 11 JULY 1979

East Wylie Street has become a real kindergarten, full of noise and cheer. The street's children, Matthew's next-door neighbor Anna, on whom he seems to have a crush, Jesse Sanders from across the street (his family just returned from a sabbatical in Oregon), attract children from other nearby areas, such as Daniel G., who lives just around the corner, on First Street. To block out their shouting, crying, and squealing, I draw a curtain between myself and the outside world, a magic curtain of sounds: these days, it's mostly Beethoven's quartets [. . .] As I look at Matthew, who people say bears a striking resemblance to me (I do not see this personally, although I do detect a family resemblance to photos of my own chubby face at two or three years of age), I try to retrieve bits of my early childhood, of my obscure pre-history, of which I have no conscious recollection. From what my mother tells me and from the round face in the old photographs, mute as archeological remains, I gather that Matthew has the same devouring appetite that I had at his age. Like him, I had a sweet tooth. (Whenever my mother appeared, she told me later, I would always shout happily, expecting chocolate.) Like him, perhaps, I felt a need to incorporate whatever was available. Matthew thrusts everything he finds in his mouth: leaves and stones, flower petals and earth, blades of grass and bits of rusty metal . . .

❋ 27 JULY 1979

. . . Poor Matthew had a bad fall, three days ago, in one of the rare moments when he was out of our sight, rolling from the top of the stairs all the way down, where, in terror and certainly also in pain, he began to scream and cry—a prolonged, frightening wailing. He seemed unable—or unwilling?—to get up. I took him in my arms and we tried to calm him down, although by then I was panicking myself. We thought he had bumped his head or broken something—doctors, X-rays, tests. But no, it was less serious than we feared, just a few bruises on his head, a torn ligament, a sprained ankle. The fact is, from that moment on, he stopped walking, and reverted to crawling about on all fours. Today, when Uca picked me up at the airport in Indianapolis, I found her as worried as when I had left the previous day for Buffalo (where I was invited, with Raymond Federman and Ihab Hassan, to participate in a conference on postmodernism); she was as worried as she sounded last night on the phone, and the tone of her voice was as sad. We took Matthew to the doctor again, and then back to the X-ray department. They found nothing, I'm happy to say. But the poor child, temporarily unable to expend his energy as he did before the accident, is a bit nervous. Probably everything will be OK in a few days.

❋ 12 AUGUST 1979

We went, Uca, myself, and Matthew (I carried him on my back for two long, tiring hours, but what a sweet burden) on the "big circle" in Brown County. It is one of our favorite hikes,.through a forest that encircles a marshy extension of Lake Monroe, a reserve for migrating birds, a stopover on their long-haul flights. What wonderful air, what blending of scents after yesterday's rain: flowers and last year's rotting leaves! [. . .] Matthew, delightful, cheerfully expansive, after about two weeks of "brooding," during which he has been walking on all fours, and then limping for a while, probably vividly remembering his tumble down the stairs. He is now fully recovered, and blooming in his childish "anarchism." That the term anarchism is entirely appropriate in his case is proved by his whole attitude toward "authority" (i.e., us) and toward family authoritarianism. And because we love him and understand him, his anarchism is cheerful, jolly, likeable. Nothing amuses him more than interdictions, than being told "Don't do that." "Don't do that" sounds at once so funny and amazing to him that he actually stops doing whatever it was that he was doing (it is one of his signature pranks) and bursts out in loud peals of laughter, telling me or Uca: "Don't do that, Dad!" "Don't do that, Mom!" and then shouts louder and louder: "No, no, no, no," in a sort of verbal game of echoes and echoes-within-echoes, in a contagious playful crescendo that pulverizes all attempts at "authoritarianism" on our part. So, between the three of us, "Don't do that!" has become a private joke, the words have lost their proper meaning and have become . . . an invitation to play. Whenever I see him looking bored, unoccupied, not knowing what to do, I utter the magic formula and he cheers up instantly, throwing the words back at me, laughing heartily and all set to play. In his turn, if he sees me worried or thoughtful (or is simply keen to play), he starts shouting at me out of the blue: "Don't do that, Dad!" which seems to suggest that I have to cheer up instantly and play with him . . .

❋ 19 AUGUST 1979

What surprises me in Matthew is how much earlier he has developed the negative function of language as opposed to the positive. "No" precedes "Yes," an almost philosophic proposition. "No" seems to come from our depths, while "Yes" appears as a concession, an acceptance, an act of submission. I almost feel tempted to write an essay on the primordial character of "No." Anyway, a few days before his second birthday, he seems unwilling to say "Yes." Instead of "Yes" (when it is appropriate, when he likes whatever I suggest to him) he prefers replying by repeating my whole question in the affirmative register. For instance, if I ask him "Do you want us to go to your room and read a story?" his usual answer will be "I want (or we want) to go to my room and read a story." This is sometimes followed by an emphatic, sometimes happy, "Yes."

❋ 24 AUGUST 1979

Matthew turns two today. Uca has bought him a few presents and a cake. The children of the neighborhood have been given party favors. Their par-

ents have also been invited, they have all gathered, chatting, in the backyard. When the "solemn" moment arrives and I light the party candles
stuck in the cake, Matthew places his palms over his ears (a sign that he is
scared, but why?) and, holding back his tears, almost runs away. I hold him,
but there is no way of convincing him to blow the candles out. "No, no, no."
The other children urge him on, we all sing "Happy Birthday" three times,
but he sits motionless in front of the candles which, however, are suddenly,
and to his great joy, extinguished by a breath of wind. We then take a few
pictures, but the camera flash frightens him too, and he starts crying—he
seems to have formed a kind of phobia of fire and strong flashes of light,
after the scare of last week's violent thunderstorms. (Was it because he associated the fire on the candles with the lightning and the deafening thunder claps that he covered his ears?) After that difficult moment, he becomes
himself again: sweet, strong, energetic and communicative (he speaks well,
occasionally mixing English and Romanian, the latter acquired from the
endearments of his mother and of his two visiting grandmothers). The
party has long been over, it is now dark, but I must interrupt this entry,
because Matthew has just stormed into my study, shouting: "Don't do that,
Dad!" and hitting my electric typewriter with both fists, although I was
not even using it, since I was writing instead in longhand with a ballpoint
pen. I have to stop, I must save the typewriter, it's only two weeks since I
had it repaired.

✽ 9 SEPTEMBER 1979 (SUNDAY)

I had a wonderful walk in Bryan Park with Matthew, we ran around in
the freshly mowed grass, the almost alpine air was charged with the smell
of fresh hay, we stopped in the playground, which was deserted in spite of
the nice weather. We had a go on the merry-go-round, then Matthew rode
a carousel-horse, the rusty coils of which screeched in the surrounding
silence, interrupted occasionally by the happy barking of some dog allowed
to run freely. The barking of those happy dogs still resonates in my ears: it
is possibly the most readily identifiable sonorous signal of happiness. An
immense, almost overwhelming, sense of peace . . .

✳ 11 SEPTEMBER 1979

The linguistic tribulations, the inexpressible emotional torments of exile. With Matthew I talk mainly in English and with Uca mainly in Romanian. I am painfully aware that I lack many of the words and expressions of that emotive vocabulary that a parent uses spontaneously to communicate with a child. And not only the vocabulary, but also the inflections, the tonality, the music. I try to compensate by reading to him aloud every evening from a large illustrated edition of Mother Goose nursery rhymes. And, amazingly, although I am aware that my voice doesn't sound right, he enjoys it. He has even learned by heart a few of those short semi-absurd poems, starting with Humpty Dumpty. Who is Humpty Dumpty? I ask him. He knows and answers laughing: "An egg, an egg that falls and breaks!"

Chapter Two

"Anyone's Death Is a Great Tragedy"

TWO DAYS AFTER MATTHEW suddenly stopped breathing during an epileptic seizure, I had the following imaginary exchange with him: "Your death is a great tragedy for us." "Anyone's death is a great tragedy," he replied. That was his way of thinking. Not his own death as an individual, but death in general, everyone's death, was the great tragedy. But it was also a thoroughly banal tragedy, like any other predictable event, no matter how terrible. And such things—it was an old conviction of his—were hardly worth talking about. His response held an underlying meaning, precisely because it was far removed from any personal context, because it had nothing to do with him, with us, because it was a known, if painful, truth, terrifying in a kind of abstract way, but above all, *known*—once and for all time. The underlying meaning, with a hint of the polemical, was this: "Let's not talk about it, it's old news, what's the point of going on about it."

Throughout his life, frequently repeated words and phrases annoyed and sometimes even angered him. To him, they were simply repetitions, empty and pointless. He did not realize that banalities can serve as conventional signs of mutual recognition and goodwill, as social indicators that communication, if needed, is welcome—with the tacit understanding that, in many cases, it is not really necessary. His aversion to the formulaic included even polite forms of address, but only when they were directed at him—he did not respond to "Good morning" for instance, or did so in a brusque, irritated, and bored way, as if to preempt a repetition. Or perhaps it was because he was ill-disposed and morose in the morning—oh, not another day, with its unfuture!—for in the evenings he responded to "Good night" and even repeated it himself several times—"Good night . . . Good night," again and again . . . as if to delay going to bed for as long as possible. On occasion he went even further; on nights when we were tired and could hardly wait to get to sleep, he grew talkative and sat on the edge of our bed asking questions and telling stories in his own way—with many interruptions—but all in a state of growing exaltation, as our eyelids drooped.

But there was something else implied in his statement—"Anyone's death is a great tragedy"—that was also typical of his manner of thought. He sometimes liked ending a discussion with a generic, aphoristic, incontestable statement like that. Whenever we tried to make him understand the differences between himself and other children—or later, other teenagers or young adults—he would say: "All people are different." Perhaps it was his way of dealing with his difference, assuming it to be perfectly normal. People are as they are. No one can become somebody else. There was also a natural, untaught, amazing stoicism in his reply to my mental remark, as I imagined our conversation two days after his sudden death: "Anyone's death is a great tragedy." This was to say: my own death is no big deal. It is a tragedy of no importance. It is a great tragedy that signifies nothing. Perhaps it was some such truth that he was trying to communicate to me, with a certain serenity, in our imaginary dialogue. But at the same time he was also trying to comfort me, for he knew my pain. He had always been extremely sensitive to others' pain. His own he took as something absolutely natural. "All people are different" meant to him: "All people are normal; all people are as they are, as they should be."

And yet . . . When I think of him, when I survey, in random order, memories triggered by one corner or another of the house we shared continuously for twenty-five years, his image—or rather images of him at various ages, especially more recent ones—come to mind: I almost feel his presence, his awkward manner, I imagine his stumbling shuffle, his heavy step which made our wooden staircase creak in a way that left no doubt as to who was there; and I am reminded how he often called for me as "Mom" at first, although he was perfectly aware he was addressing his father, and how he only eventually resigned himself to "Dad." (His mother was the one he always meant to call, from the depth of his being, with that primordial syllable in which the repeated labial consonant "m" evokes the mother in most languages.) I remember the way he talked to me, with long pauses, searching for words that never came or came very slowly after lengthy and tormenting verbal shots in the dark, often ending in frustration and dismissal. ("Never mind. Never mind.") Today, all these peculiarities appear to me not merely as symptoms of his condition, but also as manifestations of an almost extraterrestrial inadequacy before this world, not reducible to the autism that doctors diagnosed belatedly, when he was in elementary school. He came, it seemed, from another world, bearing a message I could not decode, a mystery I perceived only as a distant, rare, strange radiance that shone upon us. Postmortem constructions? Perhaps. But this was the unspoken lesson I came to learn from him—the gift of that aura of resigned innocence that surrounded him, of the spontaneous affection he attracted like a magnet wherever he went, in which he and all those around him quietly rejoiced.

I remember that when I first heard the diagnosis—wounded in my stupid pride, in the arrogance of my grandiose dreams for my son's future, not unlike, in fact, any parent's pride and arrogance—I had fantasies for a while of the two of us withdrawing from the world and leading a strictly monastic life. Because I was not a believer, this was in effect a fantasy of double quasi-suicide, of a definitive retreat from the world, of permanent personal mortification on my part. Unlike me, I felt he would benefit from the ritual, ordered life, given the chaos that human society appeared to be for him, with its tacit and complicated demands he could neither grasp nor properly handle. I was still prey to a demonic pride and ashamed of having begotten, late in life, a disabled child whom I desperately loved and with whom I wished to truly communicate but could not. But it was also—thank God—the beginning of a long process of understanding, even if it was, in the end, only to understand that I could not understand. I had completely forgotten those early fantasies, but Uca reminded me of them. I had forgotten not only because I was now at peace with myself, but also because, in the meantime, I had made so many other discoveries.

Matthew was a being apart. One day Misty, a friend of Irena's who helped Matthew at the start of his work at the public library in Bloomington, asked him in jest for an "autograph." With a smile, Matthew wrote obligingly in his hesitant, labored hand: "Professor Matthew Calinescu." What made him add an academic title? Simple logic might have been at work: only famous people are asked for autographs, and his name alone would not justify such honor. Could he have imagined that, for this one occasion, there was no harm in borrowing, also in jest, his father's professorial title? Amused, Misty showed me the autograph and I—for what obscure reason?—suggested to Matthew that he put the word "Professor" in quotation marks. He did so, saddened, or so it seemed to me, that I had failed to go along with the joke. But why had I? Why? In fact, that is precisely what he was: a professor, not a university professor of course, but a professor all the same, a shy, discreet, taciturn teacher of angelic wisdom and of the ineffable, granting gifts of mysterious peace—priceless gifts—to all those who came in contact with him.

At home, we would often witness his suffering and his all-too-human anger—whenever he did not find the right words to express himself or when we raised our voices, which his over-acute sense of hearing perceived with an overwhelming, threatening, terrifying intensity. But elsewhere, the other half of his being, the true one, was a gentle presence under the twin sign of a visible helplessness and of a very special sense of humor, one which unlocked the gates of rigid social conventions, freeing or reviving hidden kindnesses, forgotten innocence, emotional springs once nearly dry. Matthew was, unwittingly, unwillingly, a little maestro of the absurd, of a crystalline, childish kind of humor touched occasionally by the wing of poetry. Even after ten years, Daniel Baron, his former mathematics teacher at Harmony Middle School, still remembered Matthew's short graduation speech—the most memorable in his whole career, he said. At graduation from middle school, the students had been invited to take the podium in

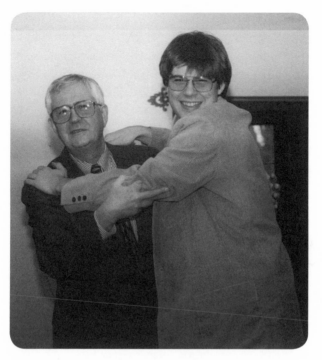

Father and son in 2000

the small grassy amphitheatre in the school's garden and say a few words each. Matthew was hesitant, intimidated by the audience of schoolmates, teachers, and parents, but finally he braced himself and, in a tremulous but determined voice, spoke the following words, recounted by Daniel Baron after the funeral at a gathering in our home of those particularly close to Matthew: "I would like to thank my teachers, who taught me many things, I would like to thank my schoolmates, who have helped me and have been kind to me, I would like to thank the school building, where I've spent four years, I'd like to thank the classrooms and the hallways, the walls and the posters, the desks and the chairs, the gym, and the garden and the trees and the bushes and the grass . . ." Daniel Baron concluded: "In fact, Matthew taught us, his teachers—and even some members of the staff who only knew him in passing—more than we ever taught him."

Chapter Three

Further Pages from the Old Diary

Today we went, the three of us, to the "circle" in Brown County: in the pure, dry air a myriad of subtle rustic aromas mingle. [...] With Matthew on my back, I climb the high, steep hill, in a kind of respiratory intoxication, in a nameless euphoria where each leaden, heavy step is at the same time the slow and, as it were, self-assured flap of a large wing . . .

❋ 22 MARCH 1980

At the age of two and a half, Matthew has discovered an ingenious way of evading responsibility for his misdemeanors: he puts the blame on someone else. "It wasn't me!" Interestingly, over the last few days, this someone else has taken the shape of an imaginary character, a bad little boy named Kim, a kind of invisible doppelganger. Yesterday evening, for instance, Kim broke a plate, spilled water on the floor, knocked over the trash can in the kitchen. The doppelganger's name is uttered with a smile which seems to encompass understanding, compassion, regret, and even a sort of gratitude. Kim is a bad and stupid boy, but no, he shouldn't be punished for his mistakes. He ran away, but will return at some point, and although he is bad, we must be good to him. We must forgive him.

✳ 7 DECEMBER 1980

Matthew is watching TV quietly—Sunday morning children's programs, *Mister Rogers, Sesame Street*. To all our other worries have been added some concerning Matthew, who appears to be going through a difficult time. He is physically well developed, perhaps a little too tall and strong for his age (three years and a few months), which may explain why he looks awkward and withdrawn among same-age children whom he meets daily at BDLC—the Bloomington Developmental and Learning Center, organized on the initiative of a few of the university faculty and staff as a day-care center for their children. Could this be the reason why, as the staff at the center believe, Matthew has started developing an incipient "inferiority complex"? The fact is he finds it difficult to do what other children in his group do (movements of a certain precision and flexibility, demanded by their games and activities, from Plasticine modeling to the little dances they do) and this gives him a feeling of separation, triggering at times silent, smoldering irritation, and even anger. A failed attempt at something will cause him to abandon it and stubbornly refuse further participation; sometimes he even feels compelled to disturb the "order" from which, in an obscure way, he feels excluded. All this has resulted in a certain shyness, of which I finally became aware yesterday at the birthday party of one of his friends at BDLC, Stefan R., the son of the mathematician Dan R. There were about a dozen other children whom he did not know and with whom he made no attempt to become acquainted. He sat silently eating cake, and afterward he played on his own in a corner of the kitchen while all the other children were swarming noisily throughout the apartment at Tulip Tree House, keen to play with Stefan's new presents, plastic cars and planes, an electric train, and other toys. All these left Matthew cold: was this self-protective indifference or a lack of interest due to timidity? Maybe he was tired. His exhaustion manifested itself after the party, when we stopped to shop at the Kroger grocery store: he started running around and, when we sat him forcibly in the children's basket on the shopping cart, he threw a tantrum, crying and screaming like someone on hot coals. Everybody was looking at us—the elderly parents of a three-year-old boy shouting at the top of his voice in the strangely muted store . . . Poor little thing: how complicated life is, even at his tender age. Complicated, unintelligible, frustrating, overwhelming. Later in life, when oblivion veils it, this age will become mythical, paradisal in his mind; in reality it is an age of trials, failures, frustrations, not of course without its calmer moments, but overall probably more difficult than what is coming next. It is just as well that it will be forgotten: oblivion is good if it frees memory from a burden—the burden of making sense of it all at such an early age, which could be much more difficult to bear than we are inclined to think.

❋ 5 APRIL 1981

In the mornings, especially after a good night's sleep, Matthew no longer seems to need the presence of a parent, the living mirror of an attentive and loving spectator for his lonely games. For instance, now—it is past nine on a rainy Saturday morning of "the cruelest month" of the year—he is playing in his room, while I in my study sip my coffee in peace, writing these notes. "In peace" is a way of speaking, because I keep the door ajar and my ears pricked: I can hear all sorts of noises from upstairs: wooden blocks being thrown, tin boxes transformed into drums, etc. These rather distant noises which come and go are not, however, alarming enough to have me rushing up the stairs to check on him. In a way, the silences intrigue me more, and make me want to tiptoe upstairs and spy on him unobserved. Over the last few days, as I spent more time with him alone—Uca and Irena were away—I managed to establish the foundations of a certain semiotic of Matthew's noises: the thud of objects being thrown, thumping on the floor, solitary exclamations and random shouts, mumblings and childish little tunes, growling and meowing, all express a wide range of feelings and states, from irritation to fury, from frustration with his clumsy handling of things, to the oppression of boredom itself. Boredom. After all, a child's paradise is seldom without its moments of boredom, and these moments can seem endless, literally so . . . I had barely finished my coffee when Matthew came downstairs asking for a drink and a cookie, and another cookie, and another . . . For Matthew, it seems to me, eating is a way of dealing with boredom or waiting around—that waiting for nothing in particular, when time thickens to an unbearable degree. Now, for instance, he is waiting to be picked up by Mechtild Hart and taken to Katy's home, where he will spend the rest of the morning with two adorable little girls from his play-group. Tomorrow will be my turn to supervise the three of them . . .

✳ 26 APRIL 1981 (EASTER SUNDAY)

Uca rightfully observes that, for Matthew, mornings are personal and sub-jective, while evenings are social. Sometimes quite early in the morning, before his breakfast, Matthew likes to play on his own, looking at pictures in his favorite books, talking aloud, and inventing words from the sounds of the languages he speaks or hears around him (English, a little Roma-nian, a little French, the bit of German he's picked up from Jeni Hart), words that possibly come from the unpredictable flux of a childish idiolect. Matthew can delay breakfast (a point when the day shifts in its develop-ment) and spend an hour, or even two, in this way, as he did today: it is a subjective and creative period that requires the exclusivity of solitude. The strange language or languages he invents may have something to do with that "private language" which Wittgenstein considered an impossibility, given the hypothesis that any language is a channel of communication; but isn't it possible that children might develop private languages, not to communicate, even with themselves, but simply to play with for the sake of the game? Are there pure languages that say nothing, turning at times into prayers that do not ask for anything? Could Matthew be praying in this way, on Easter Sunday, without even knowing it? Who can tell?

Anyway, in this early morning preference for solitude, Matthew is a bit like me. For me, too, mornings are when I have the greatest, most inexpressible need for solitude. "In the morning ideas walk on tiptoe," Nietzsche said somewhere; they float and dance in the air to the rhythm of unheard tunes, like those from the shepherd's pipes on Keats's Grecian urn: "Heard melodies are sweet, but those unheard are sweeter." For years, when I had something to write, I would awake at five in the morning, make myself a strong cup of tea (the very idea of food was nauseating) and start work in a state of inexplicable euphoria that had nothing to do with what I was writing about. Writing itself, the sheer physical act, extended this euphoria rather than causing it to abate—irrespective of what ended up on the page—and this carried me from those fresh early morning hours toward noon. The content was irrelevant, simply writing, placing words on paper, being, metaphorically speaking, at the center of a mysterious linguistic creativity, had an overwhelming subjective importance for me. Yes, I am like Matthew in this respect: but the languages he invents in the morning have no grammatical rules, he has no need to communicate, his creations are pure, totally disinterested. Now he speaks this unknown language with God's angels, and does not know it, now, on this Easter Sunday, with its dew-sparkled grass—reflecting its light back to the sun. Light . . .

❅

[This is the last significant reference to Matthew in the old diary, written before he was to turn four. I abandoned that notebook sometime in 1982, and began a journal again in 1985, the *Notebook with Black Covers*.]

Chapter Four

Mater Dolorosa

I REGARD THIS biographical portrait of Matthew as a kind of galaxy of fragments: older and more recent diary entries written when he was still alive, later comments on the margin of earlier diary entries, comments on those comments, memories, reflections, anecdotes, and notes taken while reading (always in relation to him)—all in a more or less random order. Temporally, these fragments will unfold both clockwise and counter-clockwise—as I transcribe and write. The only certainty at this point is that it all began with the end. We lost Matthew on March first of 2003, in the evening, when I found him sprawled on the floor in the room where I had left him a few minutes earlier seated calmly on the settee watching a TV program that had started at eight. It was now a quarter past eight. He had slipped silently from the settee and was lying motionless. He was not breathing. I put my lips on his, at once hot and lifeless, for a few seconds, and clumsily attempted to resuscitate him. It was like a strange kiss, intense and desperate, as I tried to suck air from his chest and then fill it with air from my lungs by a powerful, yet ultimately impotent exhalation. I finally called to his mother who was upstairs talking on the phone to our daughter, wishing her happy birthday, that first of March. Matthew was over twelve years younger than his sister.

"Matthew had a seizure and has stopped breathing," I screamed, and she immediately interrupted her long-distance call to Irena, in Los Angeles. "Matthew isn't well, I'll call you back later," she said before hanging up.

My next clear memory is of Matthew lying in a dimly lit room on a hospital bed, with eyes closed and hands on his chest, still warm as I kissed his forehead. Uca kissed his forehead and cheeks several times, and stroked his hair, crying. "If he were alive, he wouldn't let me kiss him," she said calmly, gently. It was true, Matthew disliked physical contact, he rejected kisses and embraces brusquely and recoiled tensely if even touched. "He's still warm," Uca kept whispering to me, as tears streamed down her face. It was not yet ten in the evening, so I phoned Father Athanasius Wilson, our Eastern Orthodox priest, who soon arrived (I had no sense of time: when there is nothing left to hope for, time simply evaporates). "This is not Matthew," he said, as he entered the room, "it is only his body, his mortal clothing. His soul has departed, it is no longer here." But Uca denied it, murmuring through her suppressed sobs: "No, this is my Matthew, my Matthew, my only, only Matthew." *Mater dolorosa.*

Father Athanasius said a prayer for Matthew. He told us that Matthew had taken confession and communion two or three weeks earlier. In his own reserved, shy way, he was a believer. He had a natural faith, although lately he had been to church less often because, he said, "they talk too much of death there." Recently, he had been reluctant to talk about death. When he was a child, he often asked me about it. Later, when he "knew"—perhaps more than we did?—he was keen to avoid the subject. Perhaps he associated the idea of death with his increasingly frequent and devastating epileptic seizures. "Anyone's death is a great tragedy." His own individual death did not matter, but the thought of death troubled him considerably. A few years before, when he had recovered after a particularly violent seizure and calmed down, I asked him in the evening over supper: "Tell me, do you think life is good or bad?" "That's a difficult question," he replied and fell silent. That silence stayed with me a long time and it is with me still.

Chapter Five

Pages from the
Notebook with Black Covers (1985)

❋ 29 JUNE 1985

Saturday morning: the air is still fresh and fragrant, but the sun is hot, today's going to be a scorcher. Matthew will turn seven in less than two months. He is on the sidewalk in front of the house drawing a new set of hopscotch squares in colored chalk. A few days ago, Uca explained to him the rules of hopscotch, and he listened with pleasure—he likes rules, he even loves them, for they establish a parallel world, one in which he feels safe. At first, he couldn't hop on one leg; it took a good deal of practice and concentration before he could take a few hops without losing his balance. His long flailing arms—in those instinctive gestures aimed at keeping balance—have something poignantly humorous about them: he is obviously clumsy; he has, as the school therapists say, motor coordination difficulties. It is equally obvious that he aims to play the game faultlessly to the very end; he is extremely tense and you can see from his face how hard he is concentrating. Over the last few days he seems to have made some progress, but also to have reached a limit, at least for the foreseeable future.

It is as though an invisible mechanism in his body functions well up to a certain point and then ceases abruptly. Matthew stumbles, puts the other foot down for a moment, and then hops on, seemingly undiscouraged. This morning he is the only child in the street, the neighbors' children seem to avoid him. To really enjoy playing hopscotch, he would need Uca looking on, her well-meaning pretense at sharing in the game. Lacking friends as he does, he holds her as mother and playmate at the same time. Not without some inward pain, Matthew now appears to have gotten used to the fact that the other children avoid him, that he has no friends, that his only friend day in and day out is his mother. Uca has gone shopping with N.S. to Greenwood, a bedroom community of Indianapolis, one of the world's ugliest places, but with cheaper stores and a wider range of goods than one can find in Bloomington. In her absence, Matthew has decided to draw another hopscotch layout; it is quite clear that he does not fancy hopping alone on the pavement, but the idea of asking me to join in does not occur to him, or possibly he doesn't dare ask. I am good at other, more masculine games such as wrestling or running, which we do whenever we go for a walk in the park: we race each other to see who wins, then race again, over and over!

The TV is on downstairs, there are lots of children's programs on Saturday morning (loaded with commercials, of course): cartoons—the voices float upward—and I hear the door open. Now I imagine Matthew is sitting on the sofa in front of the TV. Cartoons amuse him, but not as much as one might think. He can sit glued to the TV screen for hours, but he also might get up halfway through a film and start something else, like counting the paper money from his Monopoly game in long sessions, or he leaves to do something in the backyard or the street. I am almost sure he'll soon go out again to resume his drawing on the pavement—having lost all interest in how the cartoon he was watching a minute ago will end. At times, however, his attention seems fixed—but perhaps only because someone interrupts him and, in irritation, he chooses not to disengage. Anyway, in the evening, when he's called for supper, he doesn't leave the TV until the program ends. It's not so much the program itself that he seems to enjoy—watching TV seems to lend a certain abstract sense to time, rounding it off in hours or half hours, introducing an order into its passing. Or perhaps he enjoys what he sees in the evening, the noisy and, to me, detestable game shows where the contestants' points are shown on-screen in enormous glowing figures, although it is quite clear that he can't comprehend either the questions or the answers . . .

Matthew has gone out again, but minutes later he is back in front of the TV, although the cartoons being shown now—science fiction for older children and teens—no longer engage his attention. Nervously and impatiently flipping the channels in search of something that might interest him, he finally settles on an old black-and-white film for grownups, a Hollywood drama from the 1940s. But soon he is bored, or maybe he is just irritated by the frequent news flashes about the fate of the American hostages in Beirut, due to be transported to Damascus almost twelve hours ago but still in Beirut now, almost lunchtime here, evening there. Matthew has decided to abandon the TV for now, and goes up to his room to play Pac-Man, the miniature battery-powered video game he received last year as a Christmas present. He has reached a certain level of expertise in this game, and his scores are ten times higher than mine; he loves setting new records, but having set them, they become more difficult to surpass—hence irritability, reproaches addressed to the tiny electronic gadget, exclamations, euphemistic expletives (really bad swearwords and abusive language he overhears at school are taboo for him; if he hears me use vulgar expressions when I get annoyed, he reprimands me—"How can you talk like that? You should be ashamed!"—or he is simply mad at me, stops talking to me and storms out of the room). But Pac-Man seems to me a basically sterile game, and as I listen to the sounds produced by the small electronic box—the wheezing, whistling, pop-pop tones, interrupted at intervals by short series of bells ringing, endlessly repeating—I am seized with sadness at the sense of sterility that seems, as I write, to flow from his room, little by little filling the whole house. Should I go and stop him, take him out for a walk? He will refuse angrily, I am sure, at least at first. But I have to do something, anything, to wrest him from this intense fascination, this unbearably sterile fascination he has been basking in for the last half hour . . .

✳ 1 JULY 1985

Matthew can have angelic moments as, for instance, yesterday afternoon and evening. When he feels protected by his mother's presence at home he may choose to sit quietly down at the desk with bookshelves that we bought for him last year at the Scandinavian furniture outlet. The hidden neon tube sheds its gentle, soft glare, like daylight filtered through high clouds, and he sits down to write, calculate, solve little puzzles, draw and color, in silent concentration, in a thoughtful solitude that dissolves his tensions, fears, agitation, and especially his need to somehow fill the vacant, obsessive, oppressive time when his mother is away and he is—I will never understand why—worried she might not return. He can be similarly anxious when his mother is with him, but only in unfamiliar places: in small, narrow old stores or in vast, confusing supermarkets, where he cannot help but run in all directions, like a lion cub held in a cage that suddenly becomes so big that its bars are no longer confining, like a lion cub transported to an immense, alien space, where he can no longer recognize anything, where his instincts are confronted at every turn with disconcerting surprises that he cannot assimilate.

Matthew's miraculous transformation into angel-child takes place only in Uca's presence and only at home, and it is not even necessary for her to devote her full attention to him, a simple kind gesture is enough. This, or playing a game such as *Uno* or *Sorry!* for half an hour, is enough for Matthew to change as if by magic into a quiet, thoughtful child ready to sit down afterward at his desk with the make-believe homework she has assigned to him (now, in the middle of summer vacation!). He is prepared to sit there and cover sheet after sheet of paper with his awkward handwriting, for hours, even when she, tired as she was yesterday afternoon, withdraws to our bedroom to get some rest. But he knows that even asleep she is near, and this gives him a sense of security and calm and perhaps even of responsibility: he may well feel that beyond the "homework" and exercises he has been assigned, he has to protect his mother's sleep. Bent over the paper, in the floury-white neon light, his face acquires an expression of earnestness that melts one's heart, because it is naïve and serene and in keeping with his eight years of age; it is an earnestness at the same time grown-up and childish, a mix of intelligence and candor, in contrast to his tortured facial expressions in bad times. In those I have learned to read—beyond the apparent irritation, beyond the glazed eyes and the darting focus of his glance—a chronic anxiety reaching a point of crisis. I imagine it is this background of anxiety he attempts to fight by ignoring it, by trying to forget it, by taking refuge in the ongoing flow of TV images or in the sterile but engrossing game of Pac-Man, or when it becomes overwhelming, by angry rejection of the world around him, by adopting a disorienting attitude, a behavior possibly meant in the first place to avoid a direct confrontation with his own anxiety—uncontrollable and inexpressible—with the chaos pervading his mind and his soul at such moments.

I am thinking again of his fear of being alone and wonder whether it did not become entrenched in him five years ago, possibly on the day when he went for the first (and last) time to that day-care center where he cried constantly, feeling perhaps abandoned among strangers. He was then at the tender age where a child's memory retains powerful experiences not as recollections, but as imprints, and that fear may have been imprinted in his body like a deep wound, a wound that refuses to heal, as mysterious as some bodily wounds that refuse to heal for years, like abscesses that suppurate for years, sometimes until death, resistant to medication and even to repeated surgery: such wounds refuse to be healed, dislodged, cut out or wrenched from the body in which they are inexplicably embedded. Most minds, including those of infants, manage to assimilate negative imprints and transform them into innocuous memories. But there are frail minds that cannot do this, and such imprints become comparable to the mysterious foci of infection that dig their septic way through internal organs and out toward the body's surface, radically changing the life of the body's owner. The laws of the soul are analogous to the laws of the body, as are the exceptions to these rules, but obviously such analogies have only a metaphoric value, as the perplexities that breed them remain without answer and the questions from which they originate are simply transmuted from a language of the body to the language of the mind, or the other way around, while their enigmatic nature remains unaffected.

Whatever the possible explanations might be, Matthew's irrational fear, his persistent fantasy of abandonment—which he actually expressed only once, when he was four years old, in a way I find impossible to forget— seems to have been with him for a long time. But for how long? How? Why? These are questions that remain without answer. We were driving toward the island of St. Simons on the Atlantic coast of Georgia, where we were to spend two weeks on vacation with Michael S. and his girlfriend Janis, who was divorced and had a son two years older than Matthew. We stopped for the night at a motel near Macon and in the morning, as we were about to leave, we found that Matthew had disappeared from the room, where we had left him for just a few minutes—I was checking out at reception and Uca was at the car, parked some distance away, looking for something in the trunk. We thought he had just left the room and was probably not far away. We started calling his name, searching with growing concern in the corridors and the corner where the ice-maker and Coca-Cola vending machine were. He was nowhere, no one had seen him. Finally, as we left the motel grounds, we saw him far away, lonely and apparently confused, walking along the side of the highway, with the speeding traffic hissing past him. We ran after him, calling out for him, and when we caught up with him, he was in tears and shaking. "For God's sake, what happened?" "I thought you'd left without me!" he said, sobbing, yet obviously relieved. "How could you even imagine such a thing?" "I don't know." He went on crying for a while, and then in the car, with eyes still wet, swollen, and red, he smiled at Uca, who was hugging him and admonishing him gently: "How could you imagine such a thing? How could you?"

❊ 2 JULY 1985

Why? When? How? It is simply impossible to remain within the horizon of the present if you start asking such questions concerning your son's mental state, questions that pierce your mind like drills, that bore their way more persistently into your mind the more strongly you try to resist them. If the resistance they encounter is unusually brittle, such questions are bound to penetrate like a high-powered drill through a looking glass—the mirror of the mind—and the cracks and slivers slash the day's reflected horizon. The present becomes the scene of an unavoidable collision of future and past, of anticipation and recollection, and it suddenly shatters into a myriad of sharp splinters.

Pushed by the demon of inquisitiveness, which in the beginning wore the benign mask of a purely theoretical curiosity, I went to the library yesterday afternoon to browse through the latest issues of the *Journal of Autism and Developmental Disorders*. But once started, I was drawn in completely: I had come across a few articles that I absolutely had to read carefully. One was about a young man diagnosed with autism in childhood but categorized as "high-functioning and intelligent," like Matthew. Statistically speaking, only 1 out of 5 individuals diagnosed with infantile autism are high-functioning; that is, 1 out of 10,000 "normal" children and, therefore, as rare a case in its category as the symmetrically opposite case of "genius" on the lucky tail end of the bell-shaped curve first established by the mathematician Gauss. That young man had attended elementary and middle school and had progressed to his sophomore year in high school. As a teenager he had realized that there was a difference between himself and others, but his immense efforts at socialization were only partially crowned with success. Although he had had drug and drink problems, and was still drinking—the article implied—he had eventually managed to find work as a mechanic (an assistant mechanic, to be precise), after several equally modest jobs that he couldn't hold. But for someone with autism to be able to maintain himself and live independently was a huge achievement. At that apex of his life, he had accepted the invitation of a Yale psychiatrist to write, without help, a brief memoir of his childhood, a two-page autobiography, tortured and full of spelling errors, but genuinely human and moving to me, if not to the author of the article—a doctor with an "ice-cold" touch, with a super-specialized mind like a block of ice, killing everything alive with a frigid and dehumanizing terminology. That memoir was a poignantly stammering, broken, inarticulate narrative of a prolonged sojourn in hell—yes, hell, or to use the metaphor of the detestable Bettelheim (which seems apt in this case), a stay in a concentration camp of the mind, a daily experience of terror that is beyond words.

The other articles I read referred me irresistibly to earlier issues of the journal, and I bolted to the tenth floor of the library to do more reading. I photocopied a 1979 article about a thirty-one-year-old man with autism, diagnosed at the age of four by the discoverer of the syndrome himself, Leo Kanner. This adult was at the time of the interview about to complete his graduate studies, but he had given up a long time before on his timid attempts at socialization and lived a totally solitary life, apart from contact with his parents, the only people he saw on a regular basis and with whom he communicated in a rather impersonal way. They had rented an apartment for him next to their own home, and he visited them every evening—visits when few words were exchanged and he mostly watched TV. Television was his leisure pastime; he did not enjoy reading. I was struck again, in addition to the depressing facts of the article, by the professional detachment of its author, the total lack of empathy in the way he spoke about the young man's lack of empathy (and what would he know about that?), by the manner in which his narrative was visibly hostile to any detail of life that could have contradicted the strict definition of the syndrome, and by the manner in which he analyzed the case, its history, and the interview with the parents. His description of the case seemed to me a callous psychiatric variant of the Procrustean bed and a frightening example of psychiatric "authority" as it is perceived by the representatives of the anti-psychiatry movement (R. D. Laing).

I found myself, as Uca was to find herself later when reading the photocopy I made of the article, confronted with a disturbing paradox: the description of a case of autism from the perspective of what I would term "professional autism," which, of course, originates not from an (over)reaction to a mysterious source of anxiety, but from excessive self-confidence, from a mechanical exercise of medical authority, from a discipline-induced automation of affective and intellectual life. That was "mature autism," which, vis-à-vis genuine autism, stands in the same symbolic relation as the model asylum guardian, punctilious, emotionless, working according to strict rules, vis-à-vis the inmate. Obviously, this crude model needs instant qualification: this is an imaginary guardian, possibly less imaginary in cases of institutionalization, and an imaginary inmate; but the mere fact that they can be imagined in this way rather than in another is not without connection with the role played by the psychiatrist, a role with which he ends up identifying, which becomes his second nature, as it were. There certainly exists an underlying cruelty of the medical profession, a cruelty that can have thousands of motives and thousands of faces, some gently smiling (like the face of Dr. E.S. from Indianapolis), others earnest; but this cruelty exists, as one dimension of the inevitable ambivalence created by the doctor/patient relationship. At times—too many times—this dimension predominates, taking the form of the frigid medical gaze, of an affective void and a dehumanizing touch. The conclusion of the above-mentioned paradox: one is morally obliged to defend the frailest, the most desperate, the most helpless of mental patients from doctors; one must shelter them from those refrigerating spaces called psychiatric clinics.

❋ 7 JULY 1985

I fear I might be wrong—it is so easy to be wrong, to misread the signs that are there, to see signs where they are lacking, or to miss them altogether; yet this fear of being wrong, if left alone, can become rooted in the soul like a poisonous weed. So, trying to go beyond this fear, it has seemed to me over the last two days or so that Matthew has tentatively started to open up, to Uca in the first place. Could this be the encouraging effect of "maternal therapy" as she started applying it—not systematically, but not without method either—after our return from St. Simons, where we went again this year, this time with the R. family? We intuitively selected this therapy from the often contradictory recommendations found in studies on autism, studies we both read, turning the arguments inside out as we did so. Many of them (and primarily the work of Bruno Bettelheim, despite Stine Levy's warning that everything there is false) drove us into serious states of depression, but some (notably the Tinbergen book) at least had the merit of teaching us how to look, how to avoid rushing to conclusions, how to submit humbly to the object of our attention, and how to suspend the inevitable projections and hasty interpretations, slow them down, assign them to the realm of the provisional. We learned how to compare and weigh our readings in a discerning way, and especially how to avoid being influenced by them except ultimately, at that final stage where in any case few of them had survived the rigors of internal criticism and of validation by intuition.

There was another thing we learned from the handful of useful studies we read, namely how to get closer to Matthew and generate in him a wish for change and for "affective dialogue," with firm, yet not rigidly demanding patience, a patience that should be inflexible only in its gentleness, but otherwise flexible and imaginative in all respects. In order to do this, and to select—even if, I repeat, only intuitively—the most appropriate means of communication, we needed a foundation, a generous framework for comprehension, or at least a simple working hypothesis as a starting point. The negative effects of the absence of such a hypothesis—which could be arbitrarily chosen, almost unconsciously, but should be readily altered when disproved—cannot be overestimated. It was such effects, accumulated over time, that had led Matthew to where he was until recently, in his angst-ridden, helpless, often angry isolation, which sometimes made him lash out furiously at me, the outwardly severe father figure.

Even as we became aware of the gap between his intellectual age on the one hand, and his emotional age on the other, our—highly erroneous—tendency had been to ignore the problem: we treated him in accordance with the level of his chronological and intellectual age, that of a nearly eight-year-old boy, good at math but uncommunicative ("He enjoys being on his own, he is not very sociable," we told ourselves), a boy who needed to get a grip on himself and be forced into consciousness of his immature behavior, of his inadequate childishness. And we did not realize that, by treating him in this way (with the casual, hurried, harsh thoughtlessness of everyday common sense), we only widened this gap, only increased the tension between his two age levels, cruelly pushing the poor boy one more cycle down his spiraling social regression and estrangement. What is needed, as we now realize, is a complete reversal of our attitude, a Copernican revolution, so to speak, a drastic revision and reassessment of the empirical evidence against the naïve realism of perception. Matthew is not what he appears to be. We must understand the deeper reasons for his behavior.

Let me now return to the issue of an interpretive framework or working hypothesis. I must admit that without the readings I have been doing over the last few months, I would never have understood what now seems to me an incontestable fact: that intelligence and awareness (including self-awareness) derive their importance only from the sun of emotion, the sun of love around which they revolve like the earth. It is from this understanding that we should have started, and to it we are now returning, trying to start afresh. In other words, we should have sidelined the issue of Matthew's intellectual level and focused instead on his emotional level, we should have tried to make him see or at least glimpse his own emotional sun, through the thick curtain of menacing clouds, to encourage him to have faith and wait joyfully for those storm clouds to disperse, in time. We have started noting the early fruits of our attempts, but they are still very frail and vulnerable.

Uca now plays games with him that for years we have considered too childish for him, games of imagination and imitation, initiating him into what he lacked when he started talking (the symbolic as well as social sense of play): as a consequence, his speech developed in a strangely incongruous way precisely because he lacked an imaginative support and a living resource for plenary communication. These games initiate him into the language of affection and empathy, of gestures and gaze, of facial expressions and of signs outside the verbal system. Without this preverbal or meta-verbal language, with its apparently simple, but in reality highly complex and subtle expressive-affective grammar, speech develops an artificial independence from context. This confusing situation is equally impossible to overcome or endure, and breeds a need for similitude, for repetition (such as the various types of echolalia), for stereotypes and order at any cost.

Thus, for instance, at the age of three and a half, Matthew knew by heart Kipling's *Just-So Stories:* he was not only calmed as his mother read them out loud to him again and again but, to our misconceived pride, he could reproduce them on demand, almost verbatim, although he had not understood anything of them, as we now know. At the other end of the spectrum, his use of language for daily communication was limited to the most common and repetitive occurrences of family life, in which he could make himself easily understood, even without having to complete his sentences, and especially without having to "read" nonverbal signs and guess from gestures and expressions new meanings of known or lesser-known words. With him, everything was predictable, cyclical, according to a predigested, formulaic linguistics. As for the things Uca read to him out loud, we were blind enough to believe they were enriching his mental life and widening his horizon, whereas in fact they only passed the time, a time that, for him, was otherwise frighteningly empty.

Should it have come as a surprise, therefore, that at kindergarten and primary school he would succumb to the wonder of numbers and of elementary arithmetic? That was for him a fascinating language, totally different from ordinary verbal exchanges—if anything, the language of numbers was to him qualitatively superior to verbal language, purged as it was of the tormenting confusions of communication and detached from the bewildering contexts of social reality from which he wanted to free himself whenever possible. And we were blind enough to believe—with a joy that seemed like a reward for our enormous difficulties with Matthew in other areas—blind enough to believe that his strange numerophilia could be a sign of mathematical precocity! (Much later, we realized that he was unable, or unwilling, to translate current notions into numeric terms: little exercises such as "X went to the shop and bought seven apples and five pears, and then gave three pears to a child; how many fruits did he have left when he went back home?" puzzled and annoyed him. It was as though the world of numbers had to be protected from any contamination from the real world, as though it had to be preserved in its perfect transparency.)

But to come back to the strategy adopted by Uca for returning to the point where Matthew's emotional development had got entangled, and undoing the knot and starting afresh, gradually, stage by stage, without hurry—what are her early and still tentative results? I would say that Matthew has started to respond with love to his mother's expressions of love. It is no longer just the predominant feeling of dependency and the terrible fear of being abandoned. Last night, for instance, Uca went to the opera with N.S. and Matthew had to stay with me. Before she left, he implored her with a smile but at the same time with some persuasive urgency to stay at home and let me go to the opera with N.S. instead. And he whispered in her ear something like a secret that I was not supposed to know: "I feel lonely with Daddy." He was no longer terrified by the awesome thought that she might not return—that fear had disappeared. However, he felt and expressed his desire not to be separated from her, not to be deprived of her presence for a few hours (the hours he was going to spend with his grumpy father seemed too long to him). He did stay with me in the end, naturally, and we played Frisbee outdoors and then, when it got dark, we went in and I asked him to go upstairs, put on his pajamas, and call me when he was ready. I had promised to tell him a bedtime story.

He was very good and did what I asked. After a while, since I had not heard him call me, I went up to his room: he was upstairs, motionless on the landing, with a sad face and big tears coming down his cheeks—he was sobbing silently. I went up to him, took him in my arms (forgetting for the moment that he did not enjoy such contacts) and I asked him why he was crying. "Why didn't Mom stay with me? Why didn't she?" I told him that Uca was going to be back when he was asleep, but he knew this. What bothered him was that she was not there then, at those important moments around bedtime, and that instead of listening to the stories she used to tell him about her fabled childhood, I was going to tell him who knows what story with no meaning whatsoever. What he was missing were Uca's tales about the magical Bucharest of her childhood, about Perfume Street, about her friends and the incredible but fascinating adventures she had survived unharmed. Instead of making me sad, his big tears filled me with a poignant joy.

❉ 8 JULY 1985

Yes, Matthew has taken his first steps on the right path. Let me add a few more details. At the Bryan Park swimming pool, where Uca has taken him a few times over the last few days (water, it is alleged, has calming properties), he has managed a qualitative leap: he really swam, a development that we, by virtue of our new ethos of patience, had stopped anticipating. It was a pleasant surprise. He also seems to be rediscovering, as he nears eight, toys to which he had become indifferent over the past three years. His affection is especially devoted to a big felt monkey named Georgie ("Georgie, Porgie, pudding and pie . . .") given to him, when he was a toddler, by Ilinca J. Only now does he talk to Georgie, dressing him up in the clothes he wore as a one-year-old. He likes sleeping with Georgie, hugging him tightly. In addition, the typically autistic gestures of irritated rejection (which he makes, for instance, when he is interrupted as he watches TV, a habit that has become less compulsive lately) are more and more restrained; although triggered almost automatically, such gestures are no longer accompanied by the shrill tones of his protesting voice and tend to stop halfway through, as though he were overcome by shame, by an obscure sense of their inappropriateness. Finally, to show his gratitude toward his mother, who has surrounded him with much attention and warmth for the whole weekend, last night he sat at his desk and, without prompting, quietly completed some "homework" that she had set for him: this was his delicate way of thanking her. This pleasing behavior was in sharp contrast to the way in which, after visits to Riley Children's Hospital in Indianapolis in March, he showed his displeasure by refusing to do his real homework for school or by doing it with deliberate slowness and errors that he would not normally have made.

✳ 10 JULY 1985

Live communication is infinitely more complex than articulate speech alone: it encompasses both gestures and words, language and silence, conversation and inner dialogue, disclosing and hiding, verbal and nonverbal cues, and various combinations of all of these. In addition, the meaning of overt speech itself is inflected by comparisons, metaphors, allusions, and countless forms of ironic or poetic obliqueness. My reflections are prompted by Matthew's case: many of these modes are not accessible to him, he does not perceive them, does not see them. But he makes me, who took them for granted before, see them now.

✳ 12 JULY 1985

The zigzagging line of Matthew's behavior. The day before yesterday Uca took him to a circus performance at the Auditorium and it seems that the show—with its quick succession of acts and noisy accompanying music (of which Uca complained as well)—bewildered him. A loud unexpected bang, an explosion at the end of a magic trick, frightened him so that, as he desperately grasped his mother, he slightly tore her light silk top. During the intermission, he asked to go home. It would have been better if Uca had complied, but she felt embarrassed to suddenly leave N.S., Christina, and Andrei, who were also there. So they stayed for the second part of the performance. The outcome was all too evident yesterday: Matthew had a bad day, the symptoms of autism reappeared forcefully, and the atmosphere at home was charged with a tension that had evaporated last week. This aggravated my insomnia, which gripped me, digging its sharp claws ever more deeply into my mind and body.

※ 13 JULY 1985

Reading Clara Park's memoir, *The Siege,* about the case of her severely autistic daughter, I am struck by the similarity between the way she experienced contact with the psychiatric specialists in Boston and our own experience at the Riley Children's Hospital in Indianapolis. She, too, ends up by applying (as I did in the entry for 2 July) the term "autism" to the very specialists at the psychiatric institute where little Ellie had been examined. Clara Park goes even further when she compares that institute to Kafka's *Castle.* The comparison is not only convincing, but has the merit of illuminating a series of ambiguities in the clinical relation, especially in areas such as psychology and psychiatry. If it were up to me, departments of psychiatry would introduce a compulsory one-semester course in Kafka, and those failing it would be rejected, no matter how much technical expertise they might have accumulated. In *The Siege,* I am struck by the final conversation between Ellie's parents and the doctor at the Kafkaesque institute, which left them utterly bewildered. Like Dr. S. from Riley Hospital (who took the same amount of time, forty minutes), basically he told them nothing. Like Dr. S., he avoided any attempt at diagnosis or prognosis, refused to give any practical advice ("Do exactly what you've been doing so far"), but at the same time stubbornly refused to declare the child "normal" and, when pressed to define the problem, resorted to the evasive formula of "atypical conditions," concluding, again like Dr. S. two decades later, by saying: "But we know practically nothing about this."

Why did we take what seemed to be an honest admission of ignorance from a specialist confronted with an "atypical" case as an attempt to conceal the truth or at least as a failure to give us his real opinion (for a doctor should have at least this, an opinion)? Why did we regard his words as a prudent evasion of responsibility? Why should we have judged the doctor's attitude as a strange and unpleasant mixture of detached coldness, professional cowardice and arrogant complacency, when perhaps it would have been more appropriate to feel neither encouraged nor discouraged by his manner? The answer is quite simple: because his confession of ignorance was not set within the context of what the doctor was bound to have known (assuming that he was not a downright impostor, which he certainly was not). What was lacking in Dr. S.'s confession of ignorance, as well as in the similar recognition of the doctor seen by the Park family, was in other words any attempt to explain the reasons for this ignorance or to show what the medical community as a whole knew and didn't know about comparable cases. More profoundly, his words lacked any trace of human or intellectual respect for the people he was talking to. "We don't know anything" was, in spite of the benevolence of his manner, equivalent to "You don't know anything and it's better that you shouldn't know anything; and, anyway, there is nothing that can be done for you; and, moreover, you are unable to understand." The apparently modest profession of ignorance acquired the tacit meaning of a semi-insult, made as it was in front of worried, anxious parents who had come to the Castle from far away to seek advice.

✳ 16 JULY 1985

Bettelheim's death-camp theory of autism in children is deeply flawed. For a while, though, I believed in it, in my state of discouragement and disorientation following Matthew's blunt but candid diagnosis by Stine Levy. Unlike Dr. S., she was both forthright and respectful, and I appreciated that. She had, however, warned me about Bettelheim (I had told her I knew of his book and she had replied that he had done much harm and was totally wrong). In my pain, I suppose, I was trying to accept my guilt. Psychologically speaking, the only way to give pain meaning is to turn it into punishment. I had this need—this self-destructive need—for a dark, infernal, guilt-creating theory: my son had been marked when he was still an infant by the experience of a "season in hell," or to use the metaphor of Bettelheim (a survivor of the Holocaust), by an "extermination camp" experience. Matthew had therefore survived, but—according to the theory—continued to live mentally in that space of extreme fear. What an absurdity! Today, I find the opposite theory more credible, although basically it has no more explanatory power than the other: instead of seeing concentration camp anxiety, an arbitrary term, a personal projection of Bettelheim's, as a cause, Matthew's autism appears to me as the effect of a deeper, mysterious, biological cause. It is difficult to be specific about it, because it is of a purely negative order—it derives, that is to say, from a want, a lack. But a lack of what precisely?

Only vague terms come to my mind: he seems to lack a thirst for knowledge, curiosity, initiative, motivation. The most appropriate term for what is lacking is also, unfortunately, the vaguest of all: imagination, which is directed to the future as well as to the past (memory is the imagining of the past). "Blessed are the poor in spirit." As time goes by I observe Matthew more closely: the more I become aware of delicate, fleeting nuances of behavior, the more I believe that his apparent anxiety—nerves, frustrations, disproportionate irritations, bewilderments—is marginal in his life; *essentially, he is a serene, happy child,* but happy in the same way that the "poor in spirit" are "blessed." Blessed, though, not in a life after death, but in the here and now. This biblical phrase—Jesus said it—has acquired a very rich, precise, and highly technical meaning in my mind. The poor in spirit are, even in this monstrously contradictory world, happy bearers of the kingdom of heaven, or at least of a small piece of that kingdom, a blue patch made of numbers and unheard music. In a sense that we can hardly imagine (cursed though we are with the voluptuous and excruciating gift of the imagination), they are paradisal beings on this earth, wrapped up in their own identity-without-identity, which is part and parcel of the divine. Children with autism are perhaps among the very few mortal beings whose nature is close—and this, to us, is so very disconcerting—to the transparent nature of angels.

Socially speaking, of course, the poor in spirit are objects of derision, opprobrium, exclusion: their alien happiness, as if belonging to another world, is not the kind of happiness that a parent, no matter how religious, would wish upon his offspring. And yet: blessed are the poor in spirit. Blessed, yet so misunderstood in their happiness, which consists of the simple pleasure of contemplating principles of order: numbers, geometric shapes, pure models, Ideas, repetitions, symmetries. How strange to us, ordinary people, the autistic's capacity to see mathematically—the direct perception of mathematical entities, numbers, prime numbers, sums, and so on, without questioning and curiosity, without doubts or certitudes reached via the rigors of demonstration. Seeing these abstractions in a disinterested way, without ulterior motives. Matthew, for instance, sees, in the most immediate sense of the term, the solution to sums to the order of hundreds: I say "76 + 112" and he instantly answers without thinking, "188"; if I repeat "188" with an interrogative intonation, he starts calculating in his mind and is wrong, so he has to recalculate on paper. But he invariably sees the result of such additions, even more complicated ones, instantly, without thinking.

❋

In connection with my idea of living near to a monastery (in many ways, it is both more and less ridiculous than it might appear): life in our house has become quasi-monastic: austerity, abstinence; the only missing component is prayer. Our "social" life is next to nil: we are no longer entertaining, we are no longer invited out.

❋

I am having revelations about basic but amazing facts: intellectual distances—for instance, grammatical distances between nouns, adjectives, and verbs—are interstellar distances; pronouns, prepositions, and conjunctions belong to different galaxies. Everyday things are miraculous. Seen in slow motion, an ordinary gesture becomes a bundle of miracles. Seen in slow motion, a sentence that describes the bundle of miracles in an ordinary gesture magnifies it a thousand times: the density of miracle becomes inconceivable, truly impenetrable.

✳

Last night, with delight, Matthew discovered the game of Scrabble: letters and numbers existing in a magical surrounding vacuum, in a fascinating ludic nothingness. I had bought it seven or eight years ago, after reading Nabokov's *Ada*. However, Nabokov's passion for the game failed to enthrall me for long. What was the attraction of Scrabble for Nabokov? I think it provided the possibility of giving an occasional playful structure (in itself arbitrary, subject only to ludic necessity) to the immense verbal richness of his genius, to his fabulous multi-linguistic memory. It also became, like chess, a source of inspiration. Curiously, Matthew is also attracted to this game, as he is to chess. I wonder why? Perhaps because such games, complicated as they are, create their own context and are free, at least for someone like him, from associations with the messy world of everyday life.

Chapter Six

The Story of an Autistic Missionary

Phil Wheeler, an older friend of Matthew's and his mentor—a fifty-year-old autistic man, married with two sons—came to the house to talk about Matthew. His face was swollen from crying and he repeatedly burst into tears during our conversation, interrupting himself, repeating in a voice that was hoarse with so much talking and crying: "My heart is broken."

Fourteen years ago, when Matthew was attending Harmony Middle School, Phil offered to help him with his homework in mathematics, where he had occasional difficulties. These were principally difficulties in translating problems from the ordinary, everyday language in which they were presented in class to the mathematical language in which they had to be solved. Matthew did not understand why problems were not posed directly, without paraphrases, imagery, and concrete references to the messy world from which he sought to escape. He found the didactic and often artificial contextualizing hard to figure out, and would have much preferred to deal with mathematical questions in purely mathematical terms.

The school had contacted the Indiana Center for Autism, where Marci, Phil's wife, worked; she recommended her husband, who was unemployed at the time and available, ready to do volunteer work, and all the more ready to help a child who like himself was affected by autism. He started dropping by the school after classes, once or later twice a week, and immediately formed a bond with Matthew well beyond the duties of a private tutor. We would have wanted, of course, to pay him for his services, but our offer was met with a stubborn, almost offended, refusal. He would not accept money for something he did out of love, for Matthew's sake, but also for the sake of his own mental balance, as he explained to us. He felt it was his vocation and his duty to help someone whom he perceived as an *alter ego,* as his younger self. For as long as I have known him, Phil has never hesitated to give his time and energy, with a missionary's generosity and zeal, to other people with autism. For mysterious reasons, Matthew held a special place in his heart.

Rather short but strongly built, with eyes occasionally lit by feverish flashes and a kind, slightly frightened expression on his deeply carved face (a mobile, intense face), Phil is extremely articulate, although there is also something rather mechanical in his voice. He utters words quickly, without pauses, inflections, or modulations, and this levels out his words, creating an evenness that breaks up suddenly if the person he talks to changes the subject or interrupts with a question. Otherwise, he gives the impression that he could go on talking in the same tone for long stretches of time, without regard for the other's reactions, without caring whether he is being listened to or not, and in fact hardly aware of anything else apart from his own focus on the act of speaking itself.

His life story is as follows: he was born to a modest family in South Bend, Indiana, grew up apparently without any problems at all, or rather without anyone ever realizing he had problems. In a family with scarce means and several children there is no time for individualized, detailed observation, and the symptoms of autism, and particularly of Asperger's syndrome, can easily pass for minor mishaps or peculiarities of no consequence. Moreover, as an intelligent boy who did excellently in school, he was regarded as the intellectual in a family with no intellectual ambitions.

He was a loner, had no friends among his schoolmates, and was focused entirely on his studies. Within the well-ordered structure of middle school and then of high school, he did well and graduated with brilliant results. Graduation was followed by the shock of "falling" into the real world, into after-school social life, whose lack of structure disoriented and paralyzed him with fear. Finding himself suddenly in the midst of what appeared to him a chaotic world, he started behaving and acting chaotically. Seen by a psychiatrist in 1970, at a time when fairly little was known about autism, he was diagnosed as schizophrenic and treated as such with the most inappropriate of medications, which only made his condition worse. He started work as a car mechanic in a repair shop and, after a difficult time (understandable for a beginner, frightened and clumsy but willing to learn), he was finally integrated, within the structure of demands and obligations, into the routine of a car mechanic's work. His natural intelligence, along with the knowledge of mathematics and especially physics he had acquired in school, certainly helped. His skills improved. But more importantly, he began *orienting* himself in the small world of the repair shop and in the even smaller world of his own daily activities. He thus gained some control over his life.

But, precisely because he was competent and disciplined and seemed over-qualified for the rather basic jobs he was doing, his boss decided to promote him. It was this sudden change of routine that caused his first major nervous breakdown: he lost his grip on reality, he was no longer aware of what was expected of him, and he resigned in a moment of panic. With longer or shorter gaps between jobs, he had several similar experiences: as a beginner, he managed to acquire a precarious self-confidence, only to lose it and crack up as soon as he was promoted. He was increasingly "mad." During this period, he became the father of a daughter, from a liaison with a young woman who, however, did not want to marry a schizophrenic. The mother later married a "normal" man, while Phil, with his nostalgia for the structured life of his high-school years, decided to come to Bloomington and study physics at the university, without realizing that the pattern of student life was completely different from the life he had known in high school in his hometown. But he was lucky, very lucky, as he repeatedly pointed out to me: in Bloomington, his "madness" was finally correctly diagnosed as autism (Asperger's syndrome was still unknown at the time).

Over the years, in our conversations, Phil kept going back to what he regarded as the turning point in his life, the moment of diagnosis when he started understanding himself—including the fact that the world and human society will always remain fundamentally unintelligible to an autistic person. At the University's Center for Autism, he met Marci, a quiet, unassuming, shy woman, who worked there. She must have been impressed with Phil's superior variant of autism, so different from the condition of most of the children and young people she saw at the Center on a daily basis, as well as with his intelligence and his gift with words, something she lacked. Touched by the determination with which he had embarked on the path of study (he obtained the highest grades in math and physics), she was attracted by his open, honest, unguarded personality, in spite of his oddities and limitations, which she could understand better than anybody else. She agreed to marry him. It may well be that in an impulse of feminine generosity she meant to help him, to "save" him, to turn him into a "normal" person. I know of similar cases. I remember my former English teacher in high school in Bucharest, who later became a friend and told me about her great love for a gay violinist and musicologist, to whom she had become engaged and whom she had wanted to "save" (homosexuality was a stigma at that time); he confessed everything to her, as he too loved her in his own way, and she was ready, if salvation proved impossible, at least to offer him a semblance of social respectability. Perhaps owing to his own generosity, he eventually rejected her sacrifice and the marriage never took place. A few years later, the violinist was arrested for political reasons and committed suicide in one of the prisons of Communist Romania's Gulag.

Phil married his good Marci. Two sons were born: Jake and, a few years later, Adam. In recent years the boys grew close to Matthew and came to love him. Tears were streaming down Adam's face at church during the service held for Matthew, and Jake, a teenager now finishing high school, came to us and said, choking with emotion: "You must know: Matthew is the best person I've ever met in my whole life." It seemed more than mere civility.

But to return to the extraordinary story of Phil, the "autistic genius," as I used to refer to him in my diaries: he succeeded at last in graduating with a bachelor of science degree in physics. The most arduous, almost insurmountable part of his prolonged studies was having to take a few compulsory exams in the social sciences and in English, which also included a written test. Language is one of the areas most severely affected by autism. In many cases of so-called high-functioning autism, oral examinations are less daunting, and Phil had no problem there. But written language is totally different: the brain centers controlling writing are different from those controlling speech, located in another cerebral module which, as a general rule, appears to be more severely affected in people with autism. There are exceptions. One of them is Donna Williams—more about her later—who has been able to write her moving autobiography, probably not without substantial editorial help. But Phil is no such exception. A topic that he could present verbally with some degree of clarity (although not without the occasional break or minor lapse) would be swamped in incoherence if he were to put it down in writing. With help, he was able, however, to surmount this last obstacle.

In Phil's life, being diagnosed as autistic was a liberating, happy milestone, a real revelation, as I have already suggested. The case of Matthew was different. When younger, he would have been unable to understand, and later, when I talked to him about his autism, he remained unconcerned and undisturbed. "I am what I am, and so what?" For us, however, his diagnosis was a terrible blow. There were no clear antecedents, either in my own family, or in Uca's: we searched our memories to find any signs, no matter how ambiguous, of strange behavior in our families, and of course there were some, but they certainly did not indicate anything close to autism. The enigma was there to stay and, in time, it deepened.

At the public elementary school he first attended, Matthew had a troubled time. In classes with far too many students, and at noon amid hundreds of children in the vast lunchroom, he felt rejected, frustrated, ready to react violently when laughed at or bullied (children in groups can be cruel). When he was in fourth grade, we moved him to Harmony, a private alternative school, where he felt much more comfortable. There were only eight children in his class and the teachers were not only well-meaning—as those at public school had been—but able to devote more attention to individual children. His classmates were also more tolerant. From a lone, introverted "bully" in the public school environment, Matthew became, almost overnight, a nice kid. His oddities were now regarded as minor pranks, and his jocular attention-seeking provoked affectionate responses, gentle laughter rather than the caustic, aggressive laughter with which his peers had previously reacted to his difference. This encouraged Matthew and helped him develop a technique by which he disguised his deficiencies, surrounding them with an aura of innocent-absurdist humor. He succeeded in making his awkwardness not only acceptable to his classmates and teachers but also endearing.

His mathematics teacher, Daniel Baron, told us a little anecdote the other day from Matthew's last year at elementary school. Daniel was teaching arithmetic and he wanted to illustrate a theorem using toothpicks. He asked Matthew, seated near the teacher's desk, to bring the toothpick box over to the blackboard. Matthew picked up the box and was carrying it carefully, but he tripped on his way, dropping all the toothpicks on the floor. "Four hundred and ninety-three," Matthew declared, as he got up from the floor with a smile. This was his way of camouflaging his embarrassment, with a joke. And as the children laughed, it was difficult to tell whether it was at Matthew or at his joke. And here is another such story: after one particular year-end ceremony—followed by games, singing and plays improvised by the children, and a raffle—Matthew returned home with a huge jar of jelly beans. "I won it at the raffle," he announced with a smile, "I made the closest guess for the number of jelly beans in the jar. My guess was 1,882 and there were 1,885." He took amused pride in such small victories.

In the new relaxed and tolerant atmosphere at Harmony he made rapid progress—small steps, perhaps, but important for his much-needed feelings of self-esteem among peers. In a word, he became what he really was

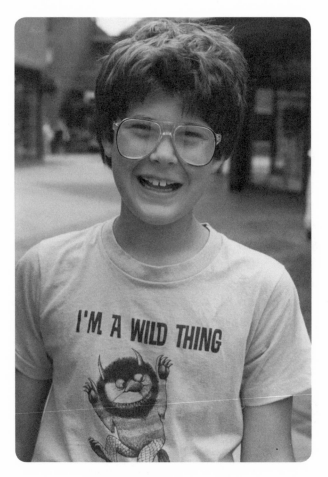

In fourth grade at Harmony School,
Bloomington, Indiana, in 1986
(age 9)

and remained: a good kid, disarmingly honest, with delicate feelings of camaraderie toward his classmates and protectiveness toward younger children, among whom he particularly enjoyed playing. He acquired a kind of gentle, naïve maturity that harmonized well with the young emotional age he retained throughout life. I gained a deeper understanding of his personality when I read Donna Williams. She confessed that, even as she wrote her book, *Nobody Nowhere,* she still had the emotional age of a three- or four-year-old, as distinct from her mental age, that of an intelligent and self-conscious adult, as shown by the high quality of her text. (It is worth noting here that, like Phil, she had had a sense of liberation when she was diagnosed with autism at the age of twenty-eight.)

We waited until Matthew was a teenager to talk to him about his autism. At that stage, we thought that perhaps he *ought to know,* although, strangely enough, he himself did not feel in any way different from others. Whenever we tried to make him aware of his difference, he invariably replied, then as well as later, with wise innocence: "But all people are different" or "People are as they are." What he meant was that what we tried to communicate to him was a truism: if all people are different, then nobody is, in fact, different. He lacked the concept—a statistical fiction in fact—of "normality." We decided to talk to Stine Levy, the psychotherapist who had first diagnosed Phil and subsequently Matthew himself, seven or eight years previously. We suggested she should have a few psychotherapy sessions with Matthew and explain to him that he had autism and what this meant. She agreed, believing that the time had come for him to *know.* But, after several weeks of meetings with him—one-hour sessions to which he always looked forward and enjoyed—she told us that Matthew was so serene, so at peace with himself, that it pained her to convince him that he had autism, that he appeared odd to others. The inner equilibrium he had attained was, in and of itself, an extraordinary achievement, and she was loath to disturb it. She spoke with genuine admiration of Matthew and thought that, in his case, therapy was unnecessary.

In the meantime, he somehow vaguely understood that he had autism, but simply didn't care: it was like knowing that he had brown, rather than blue, eyes. There was no reason for drama—or for joy. I am as I am. What's so important or serious about people being as they are? He had no reason to feel liberated or, conversely, to fret anxiously. He was undisturbed and remained so. Later, when we took him to conferences on autism, he met other young people with the same condition. He got along well with them, and with some he even became friends, carrying on interminable telephone conversations with them months or even years later. He felt comfortable among people with autism, but he felt equally comfortable among his workmates at the Indiana Center for 21st Century Scholars—where he worked for almost six years filing applications and entering data on the computer—or among those at the public library in Bloomington, where he diligently shelved books during the last two years of his life.

Matthew's relationship with Phil was of a very special order. Phil loved him from the start, he was captivated by him. In Matthew's eyes, this love was good and made him feel good because it was spontaneous and gratuitous, without any obligations—that is, free from any implied sense of reciprocity. (He hated all that was obligatory. In our family, over the years, he had managed to impose his rules: he loved us silently, without sentimental effusions, simply because he felt that way; and the love he expected from us had to be the same, unconstrained, freely given, undemonstrative.) However, a reciprocity of sorts was bound to be created between Phil and Matthew. It strengthened Phil's affection and led to certain recurring expectations. For instance it was understood that, on Sundays, Phil took Matthew over to his house, where he played games (video games, usually, but also Monopoly, of which Matthew had been fond since childhood) with Adam and Jake. On occasion they had long conversations, serious or less serious, as when Phil took Matthew out to lunch in town. In spite of the difference in age, they seemed to communicate with ease and pleasure.

Sometimes when Matthew was visiting, Phil got angry with his sons and would shout at them. Always calm, Matthew remonstrated with him: "You shouldn't do that, you shouldn't shout at your children. It's not nice." Phil complied instantly and apologized, and Matthew forgave him, saying: "Don't do that again!" Matthew had acquired an extraordinary authority over Phil, an authority which the latter accepted with total humility. Nothing on earth would have made Phil raise his voice at Matthew as he

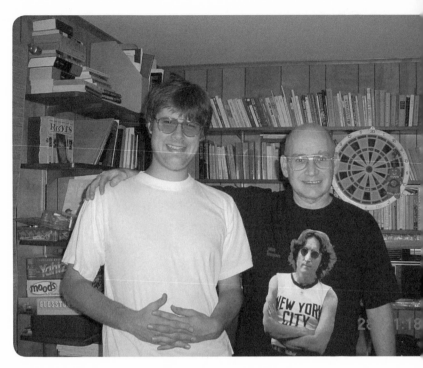

Matt and Phil, his mentor, July 2002

did with his own children. He would never have scolded him, even when he was stubborn, morose, or recalcitrant. The pain Phil felt at the loss of Matthew, he explained to us in tears, came from the fact that the source from which that authority radiated was gone. But not the authority itself. "Matthew was there," Phil told us, "he was there with me two days ago when I got angry with the boys and wanted to shout at them. Matthew pleaded with me: 'You shouldn't do that.' I *heard* his voice and calmed down immediately."

How can one explain the powerful influence Matthew had upon Phil? Why should Phil have felt, as he insisted he did, that he was *indebted* to Matthew, when the opposite seemed to be the case? What gave him the feeling that owing exclusively to his relationship with Matthew, he was more in control, more mentally balanced, eventually giving up medication, even marijuana, which he had used as a sedative for years? Was it a simple projection? Or was it that secret, invisible, undefinable moral quality that Matthew possessed, of which he himself had been completely unaware? Was it his kindness or his innocence—paid for so dearly, yet so freely given? I have no explanation. I do not understand why, but my heart is filled with warmth. Matthew's mentor had become his disciple.

Chapter Seven

Further Pages from the *Notebook with Black Covers* (1985–1986)

✳

✳ **17 JULY 1985**

Over the last two or three days, Matthew has suddenly entered one of his negative-regressive phases, without any apparent reason. I have racked my mind searching in vain for a more or less plausible cause. I assembled the most circuitous, subtle, speculative-analogic, or far-fetched hypotheses, only to shoot them down as soon as I subjected them to critical attention. I repeatedly came up against an enigmatic crystal wall. The modest signs of progress which I observed ten days ago are gone: Matthew is in a permanent state of irritability, rejecting indiscriminately any attempt at closeness, refusing to respond to the most affectionate of questions and admonitions other than with cries ("Nooo! I don't want to! Go away!") or with intense growls through tight lips, turning into a kind of exasperated moaning. Against my will, whenever I witness such "scenes" (disruptive, shrill, angry), I am seized by a nameless tension, sometimes by real fear, a pang of fear which, when it disappears, leaves behind a mute desperation and the sense, I would say, of emotional devastation. I then find myself in a wrecked mental landscape, reeling in imaginary dust and smoke as if in the violent aftershocks of a powerful earthquake.

✳ 20 JULY 1985

Reading about autism from the most recent literature backward—in the misplaced hope that recent publications might be somehow closer to the truth or somehow free from gross errors—I finally came across the 1943 article by the discoverer of the syndrome, Leo Kanner, in a volume collecting all his major papers about autism and infantile psychoses published between 1943 and the early 1970s. Kanner's intellectual superiority, in the context of the vast literature on autism, is striking. You can see in his writing the historical background of the European-educated intellectual—he was an émigré who had fled Nazi Germany. An attentive reading of Kanner's article brings me to the conclusion that Matthew is not suffering from autism. Kanner's criteria for inclusion and exclusion are clear and rigorous, and placing Matthew in the category of autism, albeit of the high-functioning variety, would be a mistake. On the other hand, it is clear that Matthew has a pervasive problem. But what is it? How can it be defined? Could it be seen as a "psychogenic disorder," difficult, if not impossible, to label? Kanner, too, adhered to the psychogenic criterion when he spoke about a possible parental etiology. "Frigorific" parents, intellectually competitive, but devoid of imagination, etc. The more recent theories reject this idea, placing the emphasis on a mysterious genetic factor. But Kanner's observations, the way he described his patients, the way he put together the syndrome, have stood the test of time.

✳ 26 JULY 1985

Uca, too, has read Kanner and she also believes that Matthew does not have autism, because he does not completely fit Kanner's criteria. His strangeness, his emotional immaturity, his apparently unmotivated awkwardness and irritations are there, of course, but his achievements, the longer or shorter periods of sweet normality, his earnestness, are evidence for a more encouraging view. Recently—possibly due to the affective and imaginative attention lavished on him by his mother—a channel of communication has emerged, a bridge allowing and even stimulating a constant to-and-fro between the two sides of his personality, the emotions of a three-year-old and the mind of an almost eight-year-old, his real age, capable of performing complex linguistic and arithmetical operations, but almost always outside a social context. I may not be mistaken when I see evidence of this interior bridging of his emotional and intellectual age in the educational game that Matthew, encouraged tacitly by his mother, has invented and which he plays for one or two hours daily with concentrated enjoyment: he is the teacher and his pupils are Georgie, the stuffed monkey toy, and Bernstein, the teddy bear. He has already taught them addition and subtraction, and now he is teaching them multiplication. With a lot of patience, Matthew writes down on large sheets of paper dozens of exercises that his pupils are supposed to solve. He, of course, also impersonates the pupils, questioning the teacher with their thin voices or answering triumphantly. With a certain realism derived from his own experience at school, he makes his pupils err sometimes so that he, as teacher, may correct and guide them sympathetically, explain things to them, or even admonish them. This morning they were placed on a chair in front of the dining table. On the table were several sheets with Georgie's name in the right-hand corner, meticulously filled with rows of numbers to multiply—Georgie's homework for the day. When I noticed the elaborate arrangement, Matthew was already at Mrs. Hooker's, where he was going to stay until five in the afternoon. [Mrs. Hooker, a retired teacher, held at her house a tutoring summer camp for children his age.] Is it just an illusion when I tell myself that, introduced within an imaginary educational situation, Matthew's numerophilia (in which I had come to see the most worrying sign of autism) may lose its sterile-obsessive quality and become a starting point, a means toward communicative extroversion, a first—but so important!—step outside himself?

❊ 29 JULY 1985

Advice to myself: I must show myself the same patience I have started to show with Matthew. I must learn to take pleasure in—or at least not show contempt for—each break from the depression that has haunted me for the last years; and, although over the past few months I have been closer, as it were, to the "center," drawn to the dense whiteness of non-significance, I must learn to rethink time in terms of the future. Blocking out the future, for fear of dark scenarios, has the unexpected effect of smothering the past as well: and the present is the preferred locus of depression, of hopelessness. Man proposes, God disposes: an old commonplace. The great miracle (albeit ultimately futile, but even this futility should be regarded as a mystery) is purely and simply the possibility of "proposing," of "setting goals" for oneself. Observing Matthew helps me see manifestations of this miracle in the tiniest and humblest of circumstances. When, for instance, he phoned little Laura (from Mrs. Hooker's group) inviting her to the house—an invitation that was accepted—or when yesterday, on our return from our evening walk, seeing Daniel G. in the street, he said, "Let's play," I could not fail to appreciate the huge distance between "proposing" and keeping silent, between the openness of "proposing" (which, of course, may also mean being open to the risk of failure or refusal) and locking yourself up in mutism, behind the brittle porcelain barricades of insecurity. A few months ago this difference would have escaped me completely.

Where shall I start? Why not from the point where I am now? From this entry, from my ability to give a meaning to the simple fact of writing this diary. Instead of indulging in my old manner of "wasting time" by writing, of filling in mechanically the interstices of time's loose fabric, nothing should stop me from thinking of these pages as a means to recover my own individual future, to open up to the future, as well as to reestablish a link to the past. From this viewpoint, keeping the diary has been a good idea. This thin thread has been my only link to a possible meaning from the depth of my depression. As I reread this entry, I realize that in fact I had taken this decision to search for meaning, to invent it if need be, at the moment when I started writing, but I was not aware, and perhaps did not wish to be aware of it. Yes, I must have the same patience with myself I have started to have with Matthew. Patience is a manner of speaking: it is more like understanding, goodwill, and tenacity in keeping minor and major irritations, minor and major disillusions, to myself; it is the art of smiling; it is the capacity to constantly alter my expectations—of seeing them either in slow motion, or in fast forward mode, with the microscope or the telescope—calm, calm, and calm again. No, I haven't wasted my time writing this diary entry . . .

❋ 4 AUGUST 1985

Yesterday Matthew had a bad day. His separateness from the ordinary world, a separateness that can take the appearance of hostility—sometimes silent, somber, oblique, but many times also direct, strange, intense—assumed dramatic proportions in my mind, as his worried father. I try to calm down by telling myself that this show of hostility must be just a defense mechanism. As I learned from reading about his condition, daily life, in spite of its look of straightforward simplicity, is in fact extraordinarily complex. For us, "normal" people, this underlying complexity is usually hidden from view, easily negotiated, but for someone like him it may be incomprehensible and infuriating. I am fully aware of all this, and yet his gestures of rejection, his inappropriate words, his protests, his clouded eyes cause me pain and remain utterly perplexing. They are as impenetrable to me as my world must be to him. All my attempts at interpretation, the explanations I seek via associations and analogies, fail. Even if Matthew does not have autism (as I insist, after having read Kanner, with an increasingly irrational stubbornness), his condition, at least in its acute phases, is almost as severe.

But what pains me most, on days such as yesterday, is the deterioration of his speech. Strangely, he speaks English, the language in which he has grown up, as though it were a foreign language, a language he would be in the process of painfully learning. In a way, this lends him an air of premature earnestness: he is like a boy who is doing his best to speak a language which he has dutifully learned, up to a certain level, but who sometimes confuses the rules of grammar, forgets the occasional word, replacing it with gestures, pointing to objects for which temporarily he fails to find the corresponding words, hidden and inaccessible as they are in his passive vocabulary. (Although limited, his passive vocabulary is infinitely richer than his active one.)

But if English is foreign to him, what is his native language? Sometimes, when he is well-disposed and speaks smilingly in his stilted English, with pauses, and in a high sing-song tone, I tell myself, joking poignantly, that his native language can only be the pure music of the angelic hosts, a language he does not speak to us, knowing we wouldn't understand. Children of his age, when they learn a foreign language in its native context, learn it quickly and correctly: Irena, who was eight when we came here, learned to speak English fluently and without accent in a mere few months. He, however, seems to have learned his English like an illiterate adult forced to learn a language in a new country. He has somehow acquired the basics, but always searches for the right word and seems to avoid all idiomatic expressions, current metaphors, or allusions, in favor of a purely literal precision. His hesitations seem to come from an obscure desire for an unattainable correctness, as almost an end in itself. Matthew's verbal repertoire is that of a seven- or eight-year-old (which corresponds to his actual chronological age), but there is a marked contrast between the awkward, stumbling, hesitant way in which he handles it and the natural linguistic ease of "normal" children. Of course, they too make mistakes, but their mistakes are, as it were, part of the general linguistic system, they are, in other words, common mistakes, typical for certain age levels, social groups, or well-defined cultures and subcultures; they are mistakes with a high degree of predictability and even, paradoxically, with a degree of correctness—they are "correct mistakes," it could be said, mistakes that could at least easily be corrected, having their visible source within a generally well-functioning, self-regulatory system, with a capacity for enriching and refining itself. But Matthew's mistakes have their source not within the system, but outside it. Hence their strangeness.

The mistakes I make in English also originate outside the English language; in fact they have their source in Romanian (from which I mentally translate when failing to find an English word or phrase) or in French, which I learned before English and with which I have always felt more familiar. But Matthew is not in the same situation: he rejected Romanian early on, from the time we set up the play-group with the parents of Katy P. and Jeni Hart, when we took turns with their parents to supervise them for a few hours daily. Around that time we stopped speaking Romanian to him, so that now he can only understand the odd word. As Matthew's mistakes, hesitations and unnatural—albeit often grammatically correct—constructions cannot have their source in a previously learned linguistic system, the only available hypothesis is that, for mysterious reasons related to the way his brain functions, he assimilated the English language in an imperfect or incomplete manner, and some of the internal relations and functions of the language escape him. Could such failings be corrected or compensated for? Speech therapists still have no answers, and in Matthew's case his sessions with the school therapists have produced no results.

After this lengthy detour, let me return to yesterday, when Matthew behaved like a psychotic child. I was affected in a powerful, oppressive way. I don't know what to do with such emotions, how to grasp them, how to tame them, what weight to assign them in my inner life. They remain within me as stubborn, uncontrollable, and deeply disturbing impressions, produced by a pérsistent recurrence of a cluster of contradictory images: his beautiful face contorted by anger in the center, and around it, illuminating it with a faint extraterrestrial light, an aura of other images, his past and future smiles. Last night, having taken a sleeping pill while reading Henry James's *Portrait of a Lady* in bed, I switched off the light when I began to drift off. I was slipping into slumber when, from among shapeless thoughts, that cluster of images arose, delineated with amazing precision: the claw of madness slashing that beautiful angry face, lacerating it, bloodying it. I had to switch the light back on again, take another Halcion, and read for another hour or so, until long after midnight. It is painfully difficult to live with these images. They disappear only when the mind's horizon is suddenly covered with clouds, which instead of discharging their energy with the rolling of thunder and the flashing of lightning, melt away into a deeper darkness. Autism may be the correct diagnosis after all.

❋ 5 AUGUST 1985

I have just reread the fragments relating to Matthew in my diary of 1977–1981 [which I transcribed at the beginning of this memoir of mourning]. These pages are like poor-quality, over- or under-exposed photos of a few years ago, lacking the clear focus that I imagined they had, on the rare occasions when I took them. A ludicrous old secondhand camera handled by a bad photographer: this is probably the most appropriate metaphor for the way in which I occasionally recorded some of the moments I spent with Matthew over those years. (I took it for granted that he was developing as a lovely and beloved, healthy, perfectly normal child, not without, of course, the occasional frustration or tantrum, about which one need not worry too much.) I can hardly find anything worthwhile now in these faded snapshots. I was not a keen observer, emotionally engaged and over-confident as I was. Love will embellish, will air-brush the small defects and asymmetries, love will always project an imaginary beauty onto the observed object. This projected beauty—which the faded photos of my old diary pages have failed to preserve—probably stopped me from capturing the early signs, the ambiguities, the oddities of Matthew's behavior, which I chose to look at in a positive, encouraging light, and regard as endearingly "normal."

But those signs that I failed to notice—were they really there? Could our games of "Don't do this!" and "Don't do that!" when Matthew was two have been symptoms of echolalia, mentioned in studies of autism? As we scrutinize the past beyond what these diary pages have to say, Uca—who was closer to him throughout that period—as well as I fail to identify such signs with any precision. Our conclusion is that, up to the age of three or even four, Matthew was indeed a "normal" child. In fact, most experts in autism agree that symptoms are nearly impossible to detect before that age. And this is because, until that age, all or almost all "normal" children are autistic to a certain extent. In its less serious forms, this condition becomes observable only after three years of age and sometimes a more specific diagnosis can only be established much later. This at least is the current state of research. Matthew started displaying certain signs—the ambiguity of which was difficult to interpret—around the age of four, when he was attending the Bloomington Developmental and Learning Center. Matthew had been attending this center for over a year when the staff noticed that he was clumsy, sometimes aggressive, generally unwilling to communicate with the children in his group, and was suspected of having an "inferiority complex."

One day, Uca received a phone call from one of the instructors, who asked her if she might agree to have Matthew undergo a psychological assessment. Uca was surprised and was inclined to refuse, but the instructor insisted and said, "We are prepared to pay for this assessment," and she realized it must be important, otherwise the BDLC people would not press the point. However, the assessment had good, even better than expected, results. A team of psychologists led by Stine Levy—the local expert on autism—kept Matthew under observation for two or three days, running a series of tests. They reached the (alas, mistaken) conclusion that Matthew might have some difficulties of motor coordination, that his intelligence was that of a child two years older than he was, that the problems identified by the tutors and instructors could easily be resolved by placing him in a more advanced group at BDLC, and that his nervousness or irritability was not due to some emotional disturbance but to the fact that his mental age was more advanced than that of the children in the group in which he had been placed at the center. Stine Levy—who, a few years later in the spring of 1985, would at once ironically and sadly break the news to us that Matthew did in fact have autism—reassured us at that earlier time that all was well, that we had nothing to worry about, taking a burden off our minds.

In his fourth year, at home, Matthew was generally an adorable, good child, with shifts of mood similar to other children, with friends who came and went in a house that was always open to them. He was also "in love" with Anna ("He has a crush on Anna," Toby, our next-door neighbor, used to say, amused at Matthew's childish courtship of her little daughter). If the psychologists who tested Matthew at the time did not find any reasons to worry, I cannot but wonder: what difference would it have made if I had been more observant, if the "snapshots" taken during Matthew's first four years had been of better quality, if I had read them more exactly (that is, in a negative way, from the unlikely perspective of familiarity with the symptoms of autism)—if, instead of running away from a totally unknown reality I had faced it squarely—but how? What could have happened, if . . . ? Or, rather, what could have happened had the impossible been possible? The old, absurd question.

❊

About the term "autism." In his study *The Language and Thought of the Child* ([1926] 1955), with reference to a distinction used by psychoanalysts, Piaget quotes Bleuler: "Psychoanalysts," he writes, "distinguish between two fundamental modes of thought: directional or intelligent thought and non-directional, or as Bleuler suggests calling it, autistic thought." But for Bleuler autistic thought, ill-adapted to reality (non-communicative), tends to be essentially wishful thinking, and creates an imaginary dream world, expressed through myths, symbols, imagery. This is an extremely broad early meaning of the term in medical language.

Piaget applies this notion to designate a pure form of non-directional (non-communicative) thought, and shows that between this type of autism and its opposite, intelligence (which is always directional) there are various degrees, depending on the capacity of the child to communicate. Intermediary forms have their own special logic, situated between the "logic of autism" and the "logic of intelligence"; the most important of these intermediary forms, according to Piaget, is "children's egocentric thinking."

Piaget also deals with the problem of socialization, of social communication, whose impairment is one of the central issues relating to autism in the current medical sense of the term. Here is what Piaget has to say: "Does egocentrism point the way to a truer introspection? On the contrary, it can easily be seen that this is a way of living [. . .] that develops a great wealth of inexpressible feelings, of personal images and schemes, while at the same time it impoverishes analysis and consciousness of self. [. . .] The concept of autism in psychoanalysis throws full light upon the fact that the incommunicable character of thought involves a certain degree of unconsciousness. We become conscious of ourselves to the extent that we adapt to other people." The implication is that autism, in this extremely general and vague sense, affects negatively the consciousness of self, which develops only through social communication with others.

The current medical meaning of autism, which grew and developed out of Kanner's initial definition, is summarized in Lorna Wing's triad of deficiencies: in the domain of *communication* (language difficulties), in the domain of *socialization* (difficulties in interpreting nonverbal cues such as looks, body language, gestures in context, etc.), and in the domain of the *imagination* (difficulties in understanding simple symbolic games, of the "as if" or pretend type, role playing, an incapacity of imaginatively turning something into something else, say a stick into a horse, a tree hollow into a magic castle, a glob of clay into a cake, and so on, as well as an incapacity for initiating actions, games, adventurous searches, and the like).

But, until the age of three and beyond, Matthew manifested only some language difficulties: his speech rhythm was slow (something that Stine Levy noted in her psychological assessment) and with pauses, his sentences were generally simple and there was that sing-song quality in his voice, that tendency to "sing" his words, the pseudo-psalmodic, rising intonation and the involuntary high pitch, which is indeed characteristic of autism but is hardly unusual in a young child and becomes more observable toward the age of six or seven. So Matthew suffered to some degree from only one of the three main deficiencies that could justify a diagnosis of autism only when taken together. He liked to play with other kids, he seemed to like pretend games, he displayed imagination, for instance, in inventing someone else (Kim) to blame for his little misdemeanors.

[There had been, however, some other warning signs, which we had ignored. His tantrums, such as the one that took place in the Kroger grocery store, were unusually intense and prolonged. Then there was his attitude after his enrollment at BDLC. When Matthew was between two and four years of age, we had an arrangement with two couples of friends, both parents of little girls: each family took turns two days per week supervising all three children in their home. Matthew had blossomed playing with Katy and Jeni, well-behaved, sweet little girls. But as soon as he joined the BDLC, he became something of a bully, pushing the other children around and making them cry. This aggressive behavior continued in kindergarten and in elementary school. "When I was little I used to be a bully," he remembered later. This was a sign of frustration, a reaction to feeling rejected by his peers, whose moods and intentions he failed to read adequately. But the psychological assessment done while he attended BDLC reassured us, and even gave us reasons to be foolishly proud, as we were told that he was mentally more advanced than the children in his group.]

* 7 AUGUST 1985

After a bad weekend, on Monday and Tuesday Matthew was extremely gentle and calm at home, with none of the uncontrollable fits of temper which scare me so, for although they are comparatively brief, their emotional aftershocks for me are incalculable. I am wondering whether going to Mrs. Hooker's, who is more of a martinet than a teacher, might be good for him, or at least might subdue him a little. Certainly he enjoys going there; lately I noticed he wants to set off as early as possible, even before eight in the morning, when Mrs. Hooker's program officially starts, and if he gets up later than usual, he hurries grumpily and is ready in no time, insisting on skipping breakfast to get there as quickly as possible. Uca speculates that the main attraction of Mrs. Hooker's place for Matthew is that it offers a well-structured situation, with a dozen children of about his age, some even younger, who submit, willingly or not, to a strict and predictable discipline (reading hours, math hours, and afternoons at the Bryan Park swimming pool). And, so Uca argues, and I think she is right, Matthew enjoys being among children who, if closely supervised, unlike the children at school, will not be allowed to pester or mock him; if they do, they will be admonished and firmly put in their place, which, for him, perhaps unconsciously, is a form of protection and a recognition of his rights and of his innate need for justice and fairness. Matthew makes highly sensitive and judicious observations about fairness and unfairness.

But more importantly—and this is a small triumph for Matthew—at Mrs. Hooker's he does not feel excluded, he is not the victim of the spontaneous and cruel ostracism that "normal" children inflict upon the weak, the strange, the clumsy, or the slow in speech and movement. Perhaps this is why, at Mrs. Hooker's, he is able to submit to the rules of the place not only without complaining, but also with a certain tacit enthusiasm. There is more in this than a need to preserve a sense of self (which, by the way, people with autism are not supposed to have): it is also a genuine, strong, insatiable social need, an overwhelming desire to be with other children, a need that can be frustrated if he is made to feel—which he does not—any different from them. This is probably why, in spite of disillusions, he likes school. He was happy in kindergarten, and he was happy at the start of first grade—"I love school, Daddy!" he used to tell me on those golden autumn days as we walked to the Rogers School, a walk of around twenty-five minutes in the rustling of fallen leaves. Even in second grade, he continued to enjoy school, but he started to fear recess. His teacher, Mrs. Lewis, seemed to like him: the psychology of the average American predisposes him or her to side with the underdog, the weak, the less able, the more susceptible to collective discrimination. She told us that he preferred sitting on his own in the classroom during recess, working quietly at his desk, claiming he was lagging behind the others. Could his slowness, which has become more apparent over the past year, and which he now openly admits, have turned into a sly defensive tactic?

❊ 16 AUGUST 1985

At the cinema yesterday with Matthew to see the poetic children's movie *Follow That Bird*. He has seen it three times already. He enjoyed it this time, too, watching with absorbed attention and laughing a few times. But seeing it again did not enhance his understanding of the story, of the various roles (positive/negative characters, secondary characters, each with their individual significance and charm). He vividly remembered details, images, particular but disconnected scenes; with each viewing, the number of such remembered scenes probably increases, but the story itself seems to escape him. Or perhaps not, but every time I try to discuss it with him, he cannot retell it. I try to help by guiding him with questions and we finally manage to piece together a summary of the narrative, but this is not important to him. He remembers scenes—sometimes long, rather complex ones—but he finds it hard, even impossible, to string them together in order, from start to finish. In other words, he is unable to infer, to fill in the gaps that viewers or readers are bound to encounter in any narrative. Matthew's deductive reasoning is very good for his age, he is among the top of his class in math—and acknowledged as such by his peers, to his great pride. His difficulty arises, I think, from his inability to make what Charles Sanders Peirce calls "abductions," that is, retrospective hypotheses that work their way backward from a given situation: for example, in detective fiction, a "crime scene" can be the starting point for a series of hypotheses that attempt to provide possible explanations and untangle the knot of often mutually exclusive possibilities. Generally, I have noticed, Matthew does not formulate hypotheses, seeming to lack the necessary imagination. The film we saw together remains in his mind as scattered pieces of a partially assembled puzzle: figures, buildings, fragments of sky and landscape are all there, the picture is emerging, yet it refuses to coalesce, because that requires guesswork, and this is beyond Matthew.

I was surprised by his failure to recognize that two obviously negative characters in the movie (mean faces, nasty looks, aggressive gestures, angry words, odious acts) were in fact contemptible. To him, they were simply there on the screen, they were as they were, he neither sympathized with them nor condemned them. The positive characters he liked, they were beautiful and attractive, but possessed no moral dimensions for him. This was fiction, wasn't it? He understood that the characters, both positive and negative, were necessary to the story, but he did not seem to grasp the difference between them, that what was being played out via these characters was a moral conflict between good and evil. In the end he agreed with me. But even at this elementary level it is clear he has problems: he finds it difficult to interpret social situations, facial expressions, and body language. And another thing: he distinguishes clearly between fiction and reality—but to him fiction is purely that, it has no connection with reality whatsoever. He does not understand make-believe, what "as if" means, he is unable to put himself in the characters' shoes and participate subjectively in their actions; instead, he places himself, as it were, in the totally contemplative position of someone who believes that evil and good coexist on the same level in fiction, with equal rights. In real life he knows full well the difference between good and bad and wants to be good himself (apart from those occasions when he loses control of himself). He has an acute moral awareness that is not, unfortunately, mirrored by a corresponding social awareness.

✻ 17 AUGUST 1985

The emptiness before departure; baggage packed, papers assembled, everything ready and I still have an hour before I leave for the airport. I am going to Paris for an international congress of the comparative literature association to be held August 20–24. I've organized a workshop on postmodernism together with D. W. Fokkema from Utrecht, the papers to be published later in a volume. I've got time to kill, so I open this notebook, which I'm taking along on the trip.

I am thinking intensely about Matthew, analyzing him with love, out of love ("love as an instrument of knowledge," a theme of Max Scheler, one of my favorite philosophers, all but forgotten today). But is not analysis also an instrument of cruelty? "I must be cruel only to be kind." What Matthew lacks (but to what extent, I do not know) is a certain affectivity based on imagining others, on the ability to read the thoughts, intentions, reactions and moods of others (including their feelings for you) and to see or, more appropriately, intuit things from their perspective. Yesterday Uca took Matthew, as a former student, to a party organized to mark the ending of BDLC's summer program. A few of his former classmates, whom he had not seen for almost three years, were also present. They recognized him immediately and greeted him with joy—the joy of seeing a familiar face after a long period of time (three years at their age must feel like thirty at mine). Matthew recognized them too, and greeted them, calling each by name, but did not stop to talk to any of them. The only person he was clearly pleased to see was a grownup, Randy (I forget his surname), the center's director, who always treated Matthew kindly, as did the instructors, all of them women. Perhaps Matthew saw Randy as the sole male role model and father figure (as distinct from myself, the father he sees daily)—someone who could be a last-resort protector, a conflict-solver, by virtue of his position, elevated above the workaday petty fray. This is all speculative, of course, but it has a grain of intuitive truth. Anyway, seeing his former mates, children of his own age, meant nothing to Matthew, failed to touch him in any way. He has not forgotten them, but he is indifferent to them. Or did shyness prompt him to hide an emotional reaction? I wouldn't think so. What is beyond doubt is that Matthew prefers the company of sympathetic adults, such as Randy, or that of small children, three- and four-year-olds, or even toddlers, with whom he is invariably sweet, gentle, and affectionate, even when he sees them for the first time. The younger children seem to awaken a kind of tender-protective sense of duty in him. It is an attitude that he expects from grownups toward himself. He has only one close friend, Daniel G. His ideal world would consist of kind adults and small children.

Upon reflection, I realize that I was wrong to say earlier that Matthew lacks a certain dimension of affectivity: he is, in fact, very affectionate, but he does not express himself in ordinary ways. He does not try to imagine and respond to what goes on in the heads of small children, whom he adores as a category rather than as individuals (and whom he feels duty-bound to protect, defending their world no matter what), in the same way that he does not try to imagine what goes on in the heads of sympathetic adults (in whose presence he feels safe and protected). With us, as parents, things are more complicated; he loves us, and he knows we love him, but he seems somewhat frightened by our love. He dislikes open shows of tenderness, particularly physical expressions: embraces, kisses, hugs, even mere touch. Perhaps he does not even want to be loved, but simply protected in a world he finds unintelligible—just as he protects younger children. In a way, it could be said that he wants to love—as an act of affectionate gratitude—without reciprocity.

✻ 24 AUGUST 1985 (PARIS)

Matthew is eight today, I keep thinking about him. I talked to Uca on the phone last night from Ina's. Everything is fine in Bloomington, she assures me, Matthew is having a birthday party today and he is happy.

✳ 4 SEPTEMBER 1985 (BLOOMINGTON)

While I was out of the country, the eleven days Matthew spent alone with his mother seem to have benefited him. In my absence, Uca told me, he has been calm, well-behaved, and affectionate. We had been worried about the change of school from Rogers to Binford, since autistic children supposedly hate change; however, not only has the move been unproblematic, it even seems to have had positive consequences. At Binford, he has a teacher with a fine reputation, Mrs. York, whom he likes, and after only a few days he has memorized the names of a dozen new classmates. Yesterday he felt proud that, after a placement test, he was put in a group for advanced mathematics. His group will study fourth-grade math, although he is still in the second grade. Since I've returned he's had a few bad moments—but not whole days—and even these moments have been less disturbing than they were a few weeks ago. This is entirely to Uca's credit: she has assumed the role of supermother (recommended by the Tinbergens) and is fulfilling it admirably.

✳ 10 SEPTEMBER 1985

In the two weeks that have passed since my return from France, I have refrained from writing about Matthew in any great detail, preferring instead to observe him over a longer period. Day-to-day observations, no matter how attentive, miss longer-term configurations and wider-ranging rhythms, which can alter the significance of details and reveal trends that may not be visible otherwise. It is the difference between a photographic close-up, precise and clear, but frozen in a moment of time, and a film of longer duration that you can stop and start at any point, comparing scenes. As the last two weeks unfolded, I discovered the following.

(1) Matthew's emotional age is that of a three- or four-year-old, although he is decidedly more open, less uncertain, and more spontaneous in emotional expression than he was two or three months ago. The unswerving, powerful yet tender love that his mother shows him encourages

him to occasionally venture forth, shyly and apprehensively, from his shell. He is playing with a wider range of animal toys and endows them with well-differentiated imaginary characteristics (habits, manners of speech, and interests). At eight he is somewhat old for this type of play, which, according to psychological studies I have read, is more appropriate at three or four years of age. I don't know when or if he will mature emotionally, but for the time being it is good that he expresses himself in this way and feels sheltered. His few and casual relations to children of his own age have also improved. With Daniel G. he sometimes manages to play for two or three hours without arguing, and even displays a certain tolerance and willingness to compromise. He seems to understand that what is needed to maintain such a relationship is, if not perfect reciprocity, at least a willingness to negotiate and please the other. Daniel G. often drops by our house uninvited, or Matthew calls him—he knows his number by heart—or he goes to Daniel's house. Unlike Matthew, Daniel is highly articulate, speaks rapidly, is intelligent and spontaneous, but it is obvious that he shares Matthew's emotional age and on this basis they communicate well. Daniel does not have many other friends, although he is "normal."

(2) School is good for him. In his early days at Binford, he had problems (Mrs. York complained that he wasn't nice to his classmates, that he was perceived as a sort of bully, but I know that he only behaves like this when he is provoked, mocked, or verbally pestered, and feels unable to respond verbally). Overall, however, he enjoys school and is proud when he is praised or placed in a select advanced study group, such as math. We have hired a former colleague of Irena's, Lori Hallal, who needs the money, to pick him up at school, bring him home, and stay with him until five, when we return from work. When he has homework, he does it under her supervision. He seems to be getting along with her and behaves himself. She is a figure of benign authority and he tolerates such authority well.

(3) Linguistically, he has made progress—or perhaps he is now displaying abilities which, for mysterious reasons, he previously kept hidden. The fact is he talks more, and the proportion of communicative language (as

opposed to the language of demands and requests or simple responses) has increased. Sometimes, when he wakes up in the morning, I find him talking to himself: not babbling like an infant, but uttering complete words and phrases, possibly following up a dream. The important thing is that when he wants to say something—to make a statement, sometimes of a general nature—he manages to make himself understood, which leads to fewer linguistic frustrations now. But with some exceptions, his speech retains that unnatural sing-song quality in a high register (which resembles but is not baby talk) characteristic of some autistic people. However, some "normal" people speak that way too: I am reminded of my good friend from Romania, L.R., a highly intelligent and sensitive individual, whose tone of voice was similar. In my friend's case, it may have been an isolated autistic trait, a residue from childhood, in complete contrast to the rest of his personality.

(4) Physically, Matthew has overcome some—but not all—of his clumsiness. This is very important. Perhaps his increased physical confidence is reflected in his more self-assured behavior. His odd mannerisms, his grimaces and other bizarre tics (which he only uses at home and wouldn't dare display at school) still recur, but in less dramatic ways than before. Without these, when he is calm, he is an unusually handsome eight-year-old boy—as people who see him outside the home invariably find.

(5) Intellectually, Matthew is clearly at the level of his chronological age, perhaps even slightly above it. He knows many things and, in good moments, displays a kind of wisdom beyond his age, with elements of stoicism and even fatalism. He does not fret about his suffering or an unfair fate that has made him different.

(6) The fact that his "nerves," fits of anger, and frustrations have a clearer focus and occur less frequently, as well as the fact that I have got used to not getting used to them—as Thomas Mann says somewhere about one of his characters—lead me to believe that I am better prepared to discern their immediate causes or what actually might trigger them. The more general cause, of course, is so-called sensory information overload:

confronted with a high rate of unexpected external and internal signals, multiple demands, and new situations that cannot be rapidly organized into coherent structures, his mind is overwhelmed by an anxious sense of chaos. Matthew deals with this by throwing tantrums, making scenes, or simply being moody. While Uca generally maintains an even disposition, full of understanding and forgiveness, always calm and gentle, I grow nervous and impatient. I realize Matthew is affected by this and especially by the occasional irritation in the tone of my voice (autistic people perceive certain sounds in a cataclysmic way, with disproportionate intensity). I have noticed that when my voice includes the slightest edge of anger, Matthew covers his ears and starts moaning with his lips pressed shut, a prolonged, intense moaning probably meant to block out that particular tone in my voice, which resonates deafeningly and ominously within his entire being. Hypersensitive, he reacts instantly not only to my irritated voice, but also to sudden gestures, a heavy tread, and tense silences: then he starts flailing his arms around, stomping his feet noisily as his face darkens. He can sit tight-lipped and motionless, stubbornly mute, refusing to answer any questions, for half an hour or longer.

This could be a first category of immediate causes—with their immediate effects—for which I am personally responsible. I feel guilty and yet am unable to control myself as well as Uca does. A second category has something to do with those shifts in attention that even daily domestic life requires. One of Matthew's biggest problems is his inability to refocus his attention quickly enough or divide it according to the demands of the situation. For instance, when he watches TV or listens to music on his cassette-player and is interrupted, for whatever reason, he responds by gesturing and shouting ("Leave me alone!" "Go away!" etc.) or simply locks himself in the room. We have long since stopped expecting to share meals together as a family: we simply announce "Dinner is ready" and sit down to eat; he is free to join us later, when he has finished watching his TV program. This may be in ten minutes, or after one or two hours. His plate is on the table, his food kept warm in the oven, and when he finally arrives, Uca serves him while he eats in silence, absentmindedly. Many experts on autism have noted this rigidity, this inflexibility with regard to attention, in contrast to the ability of other children, including the mentally retarded, to shift their attention quickly and deal with interruptions. (Matthew is not, at least yet, mentally retarded, but he is emotionally arrested at an early age; and even the mentally retarded, if they are not also autistic, have abilities he lacks.)

Finally, a third category of causes for Matthew's frustrations, in my view, arises from a conflict between a typically autistic predilection for repetition and sameness and a weaker, intermittent impulse toward competition. But this conflict may only be apparent. This is perfectly illustrated by the video game he received last year as a Christmas present: on the one hand, he wants to play forever, or at least until he is completely exhausted; but on the other hand he wants to win (playing against an imaginary opponent) and improve his score each time. Any mistake means he has to start the game anew in frustration, but by then he is spiraling down a slope of negativity and makes another, perhaps even more elementary, mistake. In time, of course, he will improve—as he has improved at mini-golf, which he still enjoys—but he does not realize that in order to really learn something one must first learn how to learn (learn from mistakes, consciously, become aware of one's weaknesses and strengths, have a positive attitude when confronted with temporary failure, have patience, and not expect immediate or continuous success, and so on). The idea of competition (if only against himself) is at times attractive to him. It is even more attractive when he has a real competitor, such as Daniel G., with whom he sometimes plays his favorite video game and whose presence motivates him to win. But he lacks something important: long-term determination. He lacks a project—be it grand or small. His willpower, I would say, exerts itself only momentarily or over a very short term. The future holds no interest for him, he is not concerned with it because, in his mind, it simply does not really exist. Will he ever discover the concept of a future? And what sort of miracle will that take?

✳ 17 SEPTEMBER 1985

A bad day for Matthew. He came back from school with a note from the teacher for Uca: he had been difficult, he had disturbed the class, in a word,

he had behaved in the stubborn and hostile manner I had persuaded myself
he had outgrown. Once home, he had trouble understanding that his behavior had been inappropriate, that his teacher had not turned angry with
him out of the blue as, bewildered and confused, he seemed to believe. It
was as if he had experienced a loss of memory. My fear is that Matthew
might end up in one of those special education classes for mentally retarded children. It would be immensely sad, because Matthew is an intelligent child. Perhaps my fear is misplaced. I hope it is. I must hope.

❊ 5 NOVEMBER 1985

Today with Uca at Binford Elementary School for a parent-teacher conference, which takes place each semester. Sharon York praises Matthew for
his progress since the start of the year. Not only has he not been put in a
special education class, as I had feared, but he is among the top students,
and very good at math, as Mrs. York emphasizes. At home, too, he has been
better lately: he is no longer as tense, as tantrum-prone as he was at the
start of the school year. Generally, he is more articulate, his speech is less
awkward and is occasionally fluent, which seems to give him a certain joy.
He smiles, laughs, makes jokes, is affectionate, but remains resistant to all
forms of emotional reciprocity. When, without thinking, I spontaneously
put my hand on his head to caress him, he tenses up at once, backing away
and looking at me apprehensively, reproachfully. Yet he doesn't mind if I
pretend I want to touch him and my hand hovers above his head, a gesture
which both intrigues and amuses him. Hugs are out of the question—although when he was three or four, he enjoyed our fights, me on my knees,
and he standing, playing a game we had named "Big bear, little bear." He
couldn't get enough of it. Now, he finds all physical contact repugnant.
When friends come to the house and hug him, unaware of the situation,
he submits without protest to this social ritual, but it is a real torture for
him.

❊ 25 NOVEMBER 1985

How difficult it is to observe! Last night I spent more than an hour with
Matthew. He was on my lap dictating sentences, which I immediately entered into my computer; he was delighted to see how, letter by letter, the

luminous characters corresponding to his words lined up on the monitor, coalescing slowly into random, sometimes absurd, little sentences. All the while I registered hundreds of details (gestures of impatience, looks, smiles, grimaces at typing errors or inadvertent repetitions for which I was responsible, bewildered or quizzical expressions) and noted numerous inflections in his voice, both in the high-pitched and the lower registers, but, in the absence of criteria of selection and an organizing principle, all these micro-details remained without meaning and perished instantly like the details in even otherwise memorable dreams. Matthew, too, may notice many things, but because he fails to connect them to meanings, he forgets them immediately. Isn't this a form of life as dream? Had I to summarize what I saw and heard, one paragraph (even of extreme banality, like this one) would be more than enough. But poor Matthew couldn't do even this. For him life is a dream, in the most literal sense, interspersed with shorter or longer nightmarish sequences.

✳ 26 MARCH 1986

Over breakfast this morning, completely out of the blue, Matthew asked Uca, earnestly and innocently, with a slightly worried but largely resigned air, and what I would call a detached curiosity (he is never really curious, and he is rarely surprised by anything; he thinks, as he puts it: "If that's how things are, that's how they are"—what better way to summarize his simultaneously naïve and deeply fatalistic philosophy of life?): "Am I an idiotic person?" Could another child have called him this in some squabble at school? Uca tells him no, not at all, but not so much to calm him—for he is fundamentally at peace, quietly eating his morning cereal, as usual—as to calm herself. "But why do you ask?" Matthew: "Just asking." No explanations. "But why?" Matthew simply locks himself in stubborn, mysterious silence. Had his mother answered his question by saying yes, he would have been, I feel, equally unperturbed. She keeps saying: "No, not at all."

✳ JUNE 1986

Summer vacation. Matthew is attending a computer camp in Bloomington, and he likes being there. In particular (unsurprisingly), he likes the computer. A few days ago, he got his year-end report card, which is quite good, much better than I expected: an A in reading, a B in language, an A in spelling, a B in calligraphy, an A in math (not surprising), a B in social studies, and a B+ in science/health. He had an interview with the school psychologist, G. E. Eastabrook, who concluded that although Matthew has some difficulties of socialization with the children in his class, particularly in situations where there are no clear rules, he is not phobic or psychotic, does not have personality disorders, is not uncreative or unimaginative, and does not have emotional problems. I can hardly believe it! Sarah Gurney, the school's occupational therapist, said that Matthew appears to be dyspraxic, which means that he has motor difficulties, especially in the area of motor planning; such difficulties can extend to the level of thinking (thinking planning). She recommended a recent book to Uca, *Sensory Integration and the Child,* by Jean Ayres, which has not yet been acquired by our university library. Uca will order it through Howard's Bookstore. Mrs. York praised Matthew effusively: it seemed like end-of-year award day! This is how Matthew is regarded at school at the end of second grade.

❋

[Matthew turned nine years old on 24 August 1986. I abandoned my diary again for a number of years, then took it up intermittently, but without any significant references to him. I started keeping a separate diary only about him in April 1993, when he was nearing sixteen years of age.]

Chapter Eight

Reading and Play

When the idea occurred to me, a few weeks before Matthew's shocking death, of dedicating the Romanian translation of my book *Rereading* to him, I felt I was finally paying an old debt; I should have done it ten years earlier, when the English-language edition was published.

It was in 1984 or 1985—when Matthew was approaching eight and autism had been finally diagnosed after a long series of inconclusive medical hypotheses—that I started to look at questions of reading in my research. At first I didn't see any close connections between this and what I was learning about the painful enigma of autism. It was some time before I realized, rather vaguely in the beginning, that my new concerns and lines of investigation were in fact not so much independent as convergent, even on occasion overlapping with my interest in autism. In 1987–1988, when the outline of my academic study had acquired shape in my mind, and especially in the autumn of 1988, when I spent a sabbatical semester at the University of Chicago, I was fully aware of Matthew's disability as I started writing *Rereading* (which Yale University Press was to bring out in 1993). And I began with perhaps its most original section, devoted to the relationship between reading and play.

In the preceding years, I had read widely but rather randomly on the subject of autism. Bruno Bettelheim's psychoanalytically inspired and by then outdated study *The Empty Fortress: Infantile Autism and the Birth of the Self* treated autism as a post-traumatic disorder triggered by an early childhood experience similar to that of an inmate of a Nazi concentration camp. The author, himself a concentration camp survivor, projected this experience onto his interpretation of the symptoms of infantile autism and articulated a strange theory couched in psychoanalytic concepts. Nowadays his theory, which symbolically constructs the parents of an autistic child as Nazi executioners, albeit at the level of the unconscious, is unanimously rejected in the medical world. I found reading Bettelheim's book a harmful experience, especially so at a time when I knew little about the subject. There were other books, such as *Autistic Children: New Hope for a Cure,* by Niko Tinbergen and Elisabeth A. Tinbergen, two distinguished ethologists who conducted much research on animal behavior and applied their observations to the autistic child. The fundamental work—but at that time I was not aware of how important it was—was Lorna Wing's 1976 study *Early Childhood Autism.* I also perused carefully each issue of the *Journal of Autism and Developmental Disorders,* which contained the highly technical recent work on the subject. As I read, torn between despair, hope, and a growing intellectual interest in the subject, I reached the conclusion that autism covered a large spectrum of cerebral and psychological disorders, ranging from the most severe forms to those so close to "normality" as to be almost indistinguishable from it.

I also discovered that, leaving aside individual differences, the three psychological areas always affected by autism were *language, imagination,* and *socialization* (language problems are less severe but not absent in the milder form of autism that became known later, in the 1990s, as Asperger's syndrome). The central disability in autism consists of an individual's lack, or impaired perception, of a whole range of signals tacitly communicated by body language, gestures, and facial expressions, that enable social interaction and a proper understanding of linguistic communication—and a resulting inability to distinguish among serious, jocular, literal, or figurative messages. In 1988 I was especially struck by the almost total absence of imaginative play in children with autism of which many researchers speak. Hence my keen interest in theories of play and, closer to my job of teaching literature, in the relation of play to reading. I was always aware that these three dysfunctions characteristic of autism (linguistic, imaginative, social) were connected, but it was only later that I learned about the possible implications and causes of this connection: the presence or absence of an ability to play.

I had noticed for some time that Matthew, then eleven years of age, had a diminished imaginative faculty. Perhaps this could explain his peculiar ways of playing. I had lately observed, for instance, that in the company of two of his friends of the same age, Daniel and Julian, Matthew was beginning to enjoy games that involved impersonating characters seen on TV. (Julian was also suspected of having a form of autism, but his father, a distinguished composer of experimental music, and his mother, a talented soprano, had chosen to ignore this and to proceed as if he were perfectly "normal.") But Matthew seemed to be content to imitate them only verbally rather than construct independent scenarios, possible lines of action, and extended narratives involving these characters. Although perfectly good-natured, Matthew's imitation appeared limited and somewhat mechanical, as if the doors of the imagination remained somehow stuck. In addition, I noticed that Matthew's reading difficulties at school were due to his inability to find appropriate images corresponding to the words he read and then to connect them. What was lacking was a broader (imaginative and social) context for his reading. A failure to build such a context meant that Matthew was unable to construct the inferential bridges between the gaps that exist in any text. (A text would have to be infinite not to contain any gaps, leaving nothing for the reader to add.) Even in the fourth and fifth grades, Matthew continued to read slowly and aloud, or in whispers, uttering each word, sometimes even uttering a word twice if he thought he had mispronounced it or if he felt it did not ring well in the verbal tune that his inner ear heard distinctly. Such slowness was surely connected to the lack of corresponding mental images, but this was not the whole explanation.

His main difficulty, which I had termed "a lack of narrative sense," concerned the integration of whatever he was reading into a context, a pattern, an imagined situation, or a story with both expected and unexpected events, a story unfolding in time, in which questions or puzzles arising in the reader's mind find a solution only later in the text. Matthew's problem as a reader was that he did not know what to expect, that he could not guess—correctly or not—what was about to follow, that he perused the text without anticipations or shifts of perspective, that he processed the information only serially and aurally. In his early childhood he relished being read to aloud, but he found it difficult to summarize without help what he had heard. Could it have been that his pleasure derived mainly from listening to the words as music, and from the fact that being read to was soothing, and that he enjoyed being the focus of attention and feeling reassured and protected? Was being read to pleasurable because it helped him forget the highly complex and confusing demands of daily life and daily verbal exchanges, in which *what* is being said—and, as importantly, *how*—always cue the response? Was it possible that his enjoyment had no relation whatsoever to the meaning of the words and sentences he heard?

In 1988, as I considered the issue of imagination in children, I read a fair number of studies on child psychology. My focus was on concept formation in the mental development of children, especially as expounded in the works of Jean Piaget, the founder of genetic psychology, but I was also interested in games approached via anthropology, psychology, and cultural history. I thus reread after many years Johan Huizinga's *Homo Ludens,* as well as Roger Caillois and the critical debates around his book *Man, Play, and Games.* I also discovered Gregory Bateson, with his highly stimulating theory of play as fiction in *Steps to an Ecology of Mind.* During a short trip to Paris to visit my sister, Marina Pascot, I discovered in a bookstore a study on precisely the topic that fascinated me of late: Michel Picard's *La lecture comme jeu* (*Reading as Play,* 1986), a largely psychoanalytical approach, which I read, pen in hand, on my return flight, but which I found only partially satisfying. In the autumn of 1988, I wrote about one-third of part 3 of *Rereading*, devoted to the role of play in reading and rereading.

In subsequent years, as I continued to read about autism, I formed a more coherent understanding of this condition which, I continue to believe, is no different from "normality" until the age of about two or three and which in some cases can even coexist with "normality," understood as an individual's "normal" functioning in society, for the whole of an individual's lifetime. But the great enigma was still there. What I understand much better now—an understanding that, alas, failed to help Matthew—is the "modular" nature of mental functions, the fact that each one of them depends on several cerebral systems or subsystems, the coordination of which is revealed to be increasingly complex as research advances. Which micro-dysfunction might be the cause of autism? There are a number of theories that at least have the merit of allowing the formulation of more specific hypotheses and counter-hypotheses, for the time being unconfirmed. On these, and on my reflections around them, more later.

Yes, I should have dedicated my study of reading and rereading to Matthew from the very beginning. I owed it to him, even though he himself was never going to read it.

Chapter Nine

On the Autistic Personality—A Stray Note

8 APRIL 1993

I am rereading—immediately after first reading it—the Austrian doctor Hans Asperger's essay "Autistic Psychopathy in Childhood" (1944), published in English translation in Uta Frith's *Autism and Asperger's Syndrome* (Cambridge University Press, 1991). The distinction between what has recently come to be called Asperger's syndrome and autism proper is not uncontroversial, but, irrespective of its validity, Asperger's article is still filled with interesting ideas and observations more than half a century after it was first printed. (Although nearly contemporary with Leo Kanner's article establishing the syndrome of autism, Asperger's was long ignored because it was published toward the end of World War II, in German, in circumstances that were bound to be unfavorable to any medical publication in a language annexed by a savage, inhuman ideology. But Asperger is proof—certainly not the only one—that the language had not been completely annexed.)

The forebears of autistic children, Asperger writes, have in many cases been "intellectuals for several generations [. . .]. Occasionally, we found among these children descendants of important artistic or scholarly families." And: "If it is the father who has transmitted the autistic traits, then he will in most cases have an intellectual profession." Asperger was fascinated and intrigued by the fact that the autistic children he had seen "are almost exclusively boys. [. . .] There is certainly a strong hint at a sex-linked or at least sex-limited mode of inheritance. *The autistic personality is an extreme variant of male intelligence* [my emphasis]."

It seems to me that in the autistic individual what Asperger calls the pattern of "male intelligence" (namely: logical capability, an inclination to abstraction, an attraction for numbers and purely mathematical relations, a lack of concern for context with all its concrete heterogeneous dimensions, a lack of concern for expressive nuances that cannot be formalized and quantified, a paradoxical mix of egotism and impersonality, and so forth) is always present, but in bizarre forms which, in serious cases, can become both tragic and grotesque. Elements of male intelligence can be recognized in autism in the same way that the features of a face can be recognized in a cartoon, the only difference being that, in autism, the caricature is no longer a joke, but a living and painful exaggeration—for the one directly affected and for his immediate family. I remember that my professor Tudor Vianu used to say to me a long time ago that "madness is the measure of the risks taken by man's intelligence." These risks are easily recognizable in the caricature of male intelligence that is autism, according to Asperger. Vianu's aphorism is in a way encompassed in the dark vision I had—seven or eight years ago, when I learned of Matthew's condition—of the cruel genetic lottery we all participate in unwittingly when we choose to have children. I am certain that without who knows what infinitesimal chromosomal detail or microscopic accident in the environment, of such disproportionate effect, Matthew would have turned out greatly superior to me: he could possibly have been a genius. Statistically speaking, he would have been positioned on the extreme right of Gauss's bell-shaped curve instead of on the left.

I am increasingly inclined to believe that Matthew inherited his autism—mutated into a serious, debilitating condition—from none other than myself. As I look back at my own childhood and youth from this angle, I can discern many of his autistic traits—in all the three main areas according to which they are routinely classified (communication, socialization, imagination)—essentially the same, if in less dramatic form. I too had difficulties communicating and expressing myself; I too was, although only intermittently, asocial; and I suffered for some years from a quasi-autistic lack of imagination, compensating for the poverty of the imagery I gathered from reality with a tendency toward decontextualized abstractions. Maybe it was a form of self-cure that I didn't let my early talent for math develop, and that I stubbornly clung to my unexpected, ambitious attraction to literature, for which I did not possess, as I well knew, a natural calling. For years, decades, my writing suffered from a painful lack of expressivity, from a poverty of linguistic imagination, from a desiccated abstraction of style and an inability to play with words. Throughout this period I read chaotically and superficially, with a certain indifference to style and to verbal textures. Socially, I was gauche, rigid, reserved—I was afflicted by a strange, tense shyness that seemed to alienate those with whom I wished to have close and friendly relations.

Up to the age of sixteen or seventeen, I suffered from a curious inferiority complex: although I did quite well at school, in my mind I was good for nothing. I lacked self-confidence and it seemed to me my secret was on display for all to see, like an open book, and that anyone who read the book could only view me with contempt. The impression that others can read your mind, while you have no idea what is going on in theirs, may be an autistic trait. Having undertaken scholarly research on reading for some time now, I discern something in the fact that until late in my teenage years I read very slowly, as if wanting to commit the text to memory (but I did not, alas, possess Borges's memory and could not remember much at all). This slowness must have been a handicap in understanding the text I was perusing. I was unable to anticipate nimbly, I did not hypothesize sufficiently, and I did not think it necessary to verify the accuracy of my hypotheses:

hence my tendency to cling to the letter of the text, often missing its more subtle figurative meanings. Thus, I presented most of the preconditions for autistic introversion, and yet it never happened.

Why should this have taken place in Matthew, whose character is so superior to mine, who has an almost seraphic candor in his calm moments, who is incapable not only of doing harm, but even of contemplating it, who cannot lie? And yet I could. Matthew would no doubt have felt at home among Swift's rational horses, who were also unable to lie, but he might have been an object of suspicion, being equally incapable of despising the ugly, unclean yahoos. Matthew did not despise anybody or anything. Hence, he did not feel despised in turn. I realize now that he did not have the "inferiority complex" I used to attribute to him in elementary school—he simply could not have had it. He felt neither inferior nor superior to others. Of course he suffered when he was the object of derision and the butt of jokes, or was provoked into reacting violently, but that is another matter.

Chapter Ten

About Compassion

Lately, reflecting on Matthew's last days of life from today's perspective—the distancing, posthumous perspective where true biographies begin, always written by others, no matter how close to the departed—it seems I can discern in his somewhat lost, gentle, and remote air the sign of a fearful yet resigned expectation of death. It was as though he had seen the fleeting face of death—convulsed, chillingly beautiful, and terrifying. This is no after-the-fact projection, I can actually see it in his final photographs. He seemed more composed, more serene, more the wise-man-smiling than ever before. He may have felt weaker, more vulnerable, and tried to compensate for that weakness of which only he was aware by smiling with that tranquil shyness. Everyone who met him during his last years, at the public library where he worked or at Harmony School, which he continued to visit on occasion—not only because it was on his way, not far from home, but also because he could see his former teachers who loved him and be among children, in comfort and safety, in an atmosphere of protective and protected innocence—everyone said that he was full of *compassion*. It was the word that arose most often at church as we received condolences, and at home, after the funeral: *compassion*. A deep, unexpressed, perhaps inchoate understanding of others' hidden frailties and pains, of that universal background of suffering masked by the mundane surface of everyday life.

Georgianne, a student who had given him tennis lessons many years earlier and who remained in touch as a friend, happened to come by the evening before his sudden death. She found him—she later told us—"very meek, eager, and compassionate," shy, open, and responsive, full of concern for her personal problems. Why was she sad, he asked her? She told Matthew she had just split up with her boyfriend, Mike, the owner of an upscale tobacconist's in the mall, specializing in imported cigars. He was a heavy smoker, and although Georgianne, like Matthew, disliked tobacco smoke, she shared with Mike an overriding passion for auto racing (a passion that Matthew as a sports lover could well understand). Anyway, the age gap between them was too great, she explained, and although Mike tried not to smoke around her, things had taken a turn for the worse and misunderstandings had come up during a recent vacation in Florida. Matthew tried to comfort her, sensitive as well to the timing of the separation: "I am so sorry, and it was so close to Valentine's Day," he told her. Touched by the echo of this memory, tears filled her eyes as she spoke to us. From wherever he was, somewhere far away, Matthew still had his own unpredictable way of participating in these small dramas of the heart.

Over the years, Matthew had become understanding, patient, and compassionate with us, too. Whenever he saw we were working on the computer, he only interrupted to ask timidly when we thought we might finish, assuming that we would find time for him afterward. For him, who was to disappear so soon. . . . Over several days just prior to his death, Uca was preparing for a lecture, reading, searching for the pictures of Greek vases she was to speak on, typing in her little study crammed with art books and magazines. I would see Matthew standing silently at her door, looking at her, contemplating her, it seemed, for long stretches of time, then tiptoeing away, making a huge effort to do so silently, because his tread was always heavy on the creaking old floors of our house. He then descended the stairs, trying to make as little noise as possible. I had never seen him more discreet, more considerate, more compliant.

The last time Uca saw him alive, on that evening of March first, 2003, a few minutes before his death, as she was about to phone Irena and wish her happy birthday, it seems to me he made an anticipatory gesture of compassion—perhaps he wanted to protect her, to reassure her, to allay any fears she might have. But what had happened? "Mom, Mom, come here!" Matthew had called several times from the TV room. Uca went quickly, not unduly worried, because it was normal for him to call to her like that. She found him sprawled on the futon mattress next to the sofa where he usually sat when he watched TV. He was lying face downward, with his head in his hands, as if deep in thought in that odd position. "What's the matter? Why are you on the floor? Did you have a seizure?" she asked, suddenly anxious. "No," he said, with a smile on his face, "you know I sometimes like to lie down this way." "But why did you call me?" "It doesn't matter, never mind!" he answered, getting up from the futon and sitting on the sofa. These were to be his last words. He kept smiling and turned his attention back to the TV screen—perhaps ten minutes before the fatal seizure.

Reassured by his apparently normal demeanor, Uca left to answer the phone, which had started ringing: it was Irena, back from a visit to the Los Angeles botanical garden with baby Rory, responding to the messages we had left on her answering machine. Uca took the cordless phone and went upstairs to our bedroom to speak with her a while in private, after which she would pass Irena on to me and Matthew to wish her happy birthday. But shortly afterward, as I went to tell Matthew it would soon be his turn to talk to his sister, I found him lying on the floor, not breathing. He may not have been aware of what was going to happen when he fell off the sofa the first time, twenty or fifteen minutes earlier, and called his mother. Or had he sensed something? Did he make a semi-conscious, final gesture of reassurance and smiling compassion? At any rate, it was his last message: a smiling, perhaps secretly melancholy "It doesn't matter. Never mind." Uca blamed herself for not having stayed with him after he called, thinking that she might have helped him, that she might have somehow prevented the seizure that killed him. But his death was instantaneous, beyond human action to prevent.

Compassion presupposes understanding, sympathy, sensing someone else's pains and concerns, sharing the visible or invisible past, present, and future sufferings of others—all of which is generally considered impossible for people with autism. I think this is simply false. Matthew belied this received opinion. All those who talked about him said he was filled with compassion—the frequency with which they used this word was striking. Could they all have been mistaken, all these different people, encountered in varying circumstances and all saying the same thing, albeit with various nuances? It is difficult to believe that these were mere attempts to console bereaved parents.

Chapter Eleven

Ages 16 to 20, from *Diary about Matthew* (1993–1997)

I have decided from this point on to transcribe selections from *Diary about Matthew*—observations, minor incidents, reflections, notes from reading—without specifying the dates, which, I think, have lost their relevance in the meantime. Between 1993 and his death in 2003, Matthew grew up, graduated from high school, and was even awarded a few minor prizes—for instance, a Personal Achievement Award given to him in 1993 by the Foundation of Monroe County Community Schools and the Bloomington Central Lions Club, and the President's Education Award for Outstanding Academic Achievement, bearing Bill Clinton's stamped signature (1996). After graduating, he enrolled as a special student at Indiana University, took a couple of freshman courses, but eventually realized that academic work was too hard for him.

Matthew was still in high school when, in 1993, the epilepsy nightmare started. After the early seizures of 1990, for three years he didn't have any, and we thought the drug Tegretol, prescribed by Dr. Wisen, was working. But the year 1993 ruined this hope. During that year, Matthew had sixteen seizures, some more awful than others. They usually occurred while he was asleep, at night, but there were exceptions. In 1994 he had twenty-eight seizures; in 1995, also twenty-eight; in 1996, forty-six . . . Matthew's life was taking an unpredictable turn, and our concerns about his autism passed into the background; we forgot about Stine Levy's positive prognosis for him, although he continued to emanate his usual charm, in the various jobs he was in, up to his death, as his workmates invariably testified.

Initially, *Diary about Matthew* aimed to record his seizures in the hope that it might supply information to the doctors who saw him, by establishing their patterns and frequency as well as a catalogue of the positive or negative side effects of the various kinds of medication prescribed to him. But as it happens, in the course of writing, I allowed myself to be carried away by my thoughts and added occasional reflections on Matthew's behavior, notes on the books I read at the time, impressions on conferences on autism that I attended, and so on. Before each medical consultation I extracted data from the diary to present in an abridged form to the doctor who was going to see him; only once did I offer the entire text to a doctor at the National Institutes of Health in Washington who, I am certain, never read it. In fact, I stopped writing lengthier entries in early 1998, soon after the visit to Washington (October 1997), and subsequently I wrote only short entries recording and briefly describing the seizures and the recommended medication.

❋ Yesterday evening Matthew seemed happy: he had spent a sunny, cold, white January afternoon at Ski World, on the hills of Brown County, with his good friend Julian, and then with Phil Wheeler and his young son, Adam, they had watched a special pay-per-view wrestling program on TV, which Matthew had been looking forward to. But this morning Matthew woke up in a somber, irritable mood, like someone after a bad dream. His right eye was swollen and painful; he did not complain of the pain, but said, yes, it was painful, when we asked. As it was Sunday and our family doctor's practice was closed, we went to Promptcare, a private health center open twenty-four hours. The doctor there told us there was nothing to worry about, just a minor scratch on the cornea. We thought that maybe something, a small piece of ice or a twig, had got into his eye at Ski World and he didn't notice.

Toward lunchtime I was working on the computer in my study, and he was lying on the sofa in the same room, silently; I thought he was about to fall asleep. Suddenly, he started shaking, his teeth were clattering, and his body was convulsing in ever-increasing tremors, like waves on a stormy sea, gradually subsiding after what seemed like an infinite time, but which probably was no longer than a few minutes. Terrified and ineffectual, I witnessed this scene, caressing Matthew's twitching head and murmuring his name. I thought of calling the hospital ambulance immediately, but when the seizure was over and Matthew fell into a deep sleep, I decided to wait for Uca; she was at work but was due back for lunch any time. She did arrive soon—Matthew was still collapsed in his post-seizure sleep. As soon as he woke up, around one o'clock, he had a new seizure, possibly even more violent, during which he bit his tongue and started bleeding profusely. This time we called the ambulance and took Matthew to the emergency room. There he was, with a high fever (101.3°), lying exhausted on one of those hospital beds with wheels. The doctor who saw him speculated—and I think he was right—that he had probably had another epileptic seizure during the previous night, one that we had not been aware of, and might have got that cornea scratch then.

The level of Tegretol in his blood, which they measured immediately, was very low, and we suddenly realized that Matthew had not taken his usual dose that morning. We had forgotten to check, as we normally did every day, possibly because of our overriding concern for his inflamed eye and the rush to Promptcare. But, if he had had a seizure during the night—how was that to be explained after his nearly three seizure-free years? Perhaps the prescribed dose of his medication had become insufficient. While still in the hospital he was given Tegretol, and he was discharged three hours later. Dr. Frasier warned us that, as the level of Tegretol in the blood increases very slowly (over about twelve hours), Matthew could have another seizure in the evening. In fact, he has just had it, shorter than the previous ones, lasting only about thirty seconds (I checked my watch this time), but possibly even more terrifying than the other two. I cried, choking with fear and pity.

*

One thing Matthew cannot grasp is rivalry. A dialogue overheard in the car the other day, with D., our friend, in the front seat and Matthew in the back (Matthew has always been reluctant to sit in front). D. says, jokingly, boastfully, challenging Matthew in the playful manner which has become customary in their relationship (D. is of course aware of his condition): "I'm looking forward to our next backgammon game and to thrashing you." Matthew: "But maybe I'll beat you! It would be a shame, though . . ." D: "Why would it be a shame?" Matthew: "Well, because I'd love to win, but then I'd feel sorry for you." D: "What d'you mean?" Matthew: "Actually, I'd love both of us to win." D: "Or both of us to lose?" Matthew: "No, no way. Both of us to win, that would be so nice!"

In his invincible innocence, Matthew will never grasp what René Girard calls "mimetic rivalry," perhaps because his mind is incapable of performing mimetic-competitive operations. He would instinctively question the notion of a zero-sum game with one winner and one loser, because, strangely enough, he sympathizes with the loser. He doesn't like to lose and attributes his discomfort to the other player. In general, he does not desire something simply because someone else does, as Girard's triangular mimesis would have it. This might be why he has so few desires and is so frugal, even an ascetic of sorts. When he visits us, D. plays a game or two of backgammon with M., who is always thrilled and who simultaneously wants and doesn't want to win. He wishes both adversaries well, rather than ill for one and good for the other (namely himself). He cannot put himself in another's shoes, but it is equally true to say that he tends to place the other person in his own shoes. If he himself doesn't like losing, how could the other person? He wants his joy—the joy of victory—to be shared with his opponent. No one should be sad or disappointed. "We should both win." This would avoid the tension of conflict while the players would love the game even more, the game per se, the beautiful rules of the game and the unadulterated surprises of chance.

On a more general level, Matthew understands and accepts as a matter of course all types of rules—the rules of ethics, for instance, which he acknowledges straightforwardly and spontaneously (it is essential to be good, to do good, and in any case not to do harm), but since he is naturally good, he cannot understand why somebody would fail to respect these rules. He cannot conceive evil—he has never been visited by Edgar Allan Poe's "imp of the perverse." The wish to do harm for harm's sake, the wish to cause harm to a specific person, the wish to be superior, the desire for revenge, the wish to pretend (other than playfully) or to lie, to cheat (in order to win) are unimaginable to him—he is paralyzed by his fundamental innocence, I would say, and innocence, when not accompanied by an awareness of the possibility of evil, is an infirmity in this world.

❉

Last night, Uca and Matthew watched Zefirelli's *Romeo and Juliet* on TV. Matthew knew the story quite well; he had studied the play at school—it is true, a few years back—and had even read, with some help, one or two scenes at the time. Uca tells me that he followed the film attentively and that toward the end, in the scene where the two lovers die, as she fought back her tears, he told her with tactful concern: "Mom, don't get dramatic. This is just fiction." Where did he pick up this phrase: "Don't get dramatic?" Possibly from sitcoms he watches on TV. But the important thing is that he does not want people to be sad. Why should fiction—just fiction—make his mother cry? He wants to be surrounded by people who feel good. Sadness has its place, on stage or on TV, but not in reality. For him, the distinction between fiction and reality is absolute. Not for anything in the world would he accept that fiction and reality might overlap. That is one aspect of his literal-mindedness.

❉

I have just finished reading Donna Williams's *Nobody Nowhere* (1992), a book with a subtitle that says it all: *The Extraordinary Autobiography of an Autistic*. The adjective "extraordinary" is perfectly apt in this case and has nothing to do with advertising hype. The book is fascinating. The author is totally convincing in her portrayal of an autistic person's strange mental world—poignantly convincing, and with a rough poetic quality. How does she manage to make the "normal" reader empathize with the autistic narrative voice? (Before I try to explain, let me say that the "normal" reader of such a book would very likely have a personal or professional interest in unraveling the enigma of autism, either as a relative of an autistic person, as a psychiatrist or psychologist, or as a philosopher interested in epistemology. However, in this case, the book seems to have appealed even to the mythical general reader and has become a best-seller of sorts.) I would answer the question in two ways. First, she does so by a special quality of her writing, what I would call a heroic clumsiness in handling language, using unexpected word choices, words that are rarely perfectly fitting, but that lend themselves easily to a metaphoric understanding; and this clumsiness goes well with her brutal candor and with a strange self-detachment, an almost "inhuman" quality of tone (a paradoxically hypersensitive "inhumanity," however, sounding as if it came from a very fragile extraterrestrial). Second, she is so convincing because she has chosen a particular narrative form, a particularly appealing type of story: a story of the quest for self and ultimately for self-understanding.

This self-understanding was achieved, after devastating experiences, when the author finally learned about and acknowledged her own autism and that of other people, people with whom she shared a mysterious, magnetic language, entirely different from our own as well as from the language in which she herself writes her story with almost superhuman effort. That shared autistic language is a silent language, a kind of anti-language made up of gestures, meant to communicate beyond words, but also to defuse the fear that autistic people have of communication proper and of the habitual gestures of love, indeed of love itself (including physical love), and of the expressions of kindness and generosity used by "normal" people. (I have noticed long ago that Matthew, too, only feels good, really good, in the company of other autistics.)

The fear of love and goodness that autistic people share sounds strange and almost incomprehensible, yet this is the book's profound theme and its primary revelation. A clear formulation of this theme appears only at the end, but it is indirectly, disturbingly, tantalizingly anticipated in each of the tesserae of this mosaic-text; it is anticipated through a sense of quest, through repeated tentative attempts, through approximations which, given the logic of our culture, do not dare say, indeed cannot say what needs to be said by the forlorn autistic person. Whenever the author manages to say what she has to say, it is an incalculable personal triumph: "Love and kindness, affection and sympathy were my greatest fear. It was great that other people had them waiting for me, but the frustration of trying to live up to their unmatchable efforts only compounded my sense of inadequacy and hopelessness. Pity did nothing. Love, despite the fairy-tales, would only be thrown back and spat on for good measure" (p. 218).

Yet, in an apparent paradox, an autistic individual needs love—but love disguised as detachment, distance, and even indifference; love that expresses itself indirectly, timidly and, as it were coldly; love that does not expect any response or form of reciprocity; love that does not attempt to "help" in an obvious, conventional way, through generosity or self-denial. "One cannot save another's spirit," Donna Williams writes. "One can only inspire it to fight for itself" (p. 219). Only well-hidden love can provide such an inspiration. Not trying to make oneself loved in return, but creating that inspiration—this is how I would summarize the book's central message. But how many "normal" people would understand its strange subtlety?

An early episode from the author's childhood suggests that her mother's brutality and the entire atmosphere of incomprehension in the home was in a way welcome, because it spared her the oppressive experience of being loved, a love to which, in any case, she would have been incapable of responding: "I had begun to walk about the house like something returned from the dead. [. . .] People would ask me what was wrong. I'd paint a smile across my face and try to impersonate my version of happy. 'Nothing's wrong,' I'd tell them in as short an answer as possible. At that point I was as fragile as I'd ever been. If I had received a lot of love, I would have probably felt that it would kill me" (p. 38).

Donna Williams was certainly helped by her intelligence, which functioned properly in spite of her extreme emotional insecurity. It enabled her to play the social role of a "happy" child precisely in order to preempt any possible gesture of affectivity, and it allowed her to live on her own in peace, with her unhappiness and immense vulnerability. Her remarkable intelligence later led her to create—another heroic achievement—her two characters or personae (in the sense of masks), Carol (a conformist, chatty false self, superficial, imitative, conventional, frivolous, optimistic) and Willie (a negative variant of Carol, equally false, a perpetually pessimistic and grumpy person, always adversely predisposed toward others). These two masks, worn alternatively in differing circumstances, were designed to hide her sense of not having a real self. The author's profound feeling, as she played this social comedy, was that she was nobody, hence the title: *Nobody Nowhere*. (Is it possible that Matthew, too, might, occasionally at least, feel that he is nobody?)

The most insightful observations made by Donna Williams are those about her fear of love: they make clear, for instance, her repugnance toward physical proximity, embraces and touch, toward all the signs and symbols of love. (How very much like her is Matthew, and how long it has taken me to understand!) This fear expresses the extreme vulnerability of autistic individuals. At an emotional level, they are vulnerable because their sensibility was arrested around the age of three—so the author believes on the basis of her own experience. At many points in her autobiography, she speaks about the gap between her emotional age (three) and her successive chronological-mental ages up to the mature time of writing the book, as well as about the mismatch between her intellectual and social ages. The fact that her emotional self was arrested in its development in early childhood is borne out, for instance, by the account of her first encounter with Mary, the psychiatrist (pp. 102–110).

Later she entered a relationship with Tim, a young man she met at the university. Although even with her boyfriend she continued wearing the two masks, Carol and Willie, she noted that occasionally she felt "it was okay to feel only three years old"—because Tim, too, seemed to be not older than three sometimes. With Tim, therefore, it was possible "to establish a marvelous sense of home. It was a three-year-old's paradise. In a childlike way, I grew to love Tim and he grew to love me" (pp. 142–143). Of course, such a relationship could not last in the real world. After they split up, Donna called Tim once—out of desperation, seeking help—and he came with his new girlfriend. Interestingly, the girlfriend felt threatened by Donna, who observed: "It seemed a cruel fate that she should have been so threatened by a child's closeness, for although I was an adult I was an adult trapped in a child's insecurity" (p. 153). In the book's epilogue, reflecting on her condition, the author wrote: "I believe I was born alienated, and if not, I was certainly so by the time I got left behind in the emotional development at about the age of three. Autistic people are not mad, nor stupid. They are not fairies, not aliens—just people trapped in invisible, crippled emotional responses. [. . .] In my case, my mind knows that affection and kindness will not kill me, yet my emotional response defies this logic, telling me that good feelings and gentle and loving touch can kill or at the very least cause me pain. When I try to ignore this message, I go into what would seem a state of shock, where what's coming is either incomprehensible or has no significance. This state leads to my emotions committing suicide, leaving me without physical or emotional feeling and with a purely robotic mental response—if that" (p. 205).

Such observations and reflections help me to understand Matthew better. In his case too it is clear that there exist gaps between various types and levels of development: the chronological age, the mental (i.e., logical) age, the emotional age (which is infantile in his case too, as I noticed long ago), and the social age. What is amazing is that autistic individuals get along well, rapidly and completely, only with other autistics. Which explains the friendships between Phil and Matthew, Julian and Matthew, in spite of differences in age and temperament. Basically, Matthew, too, is "afraid of love": many times, when I am affectionate toward him in an entirely spontaneous and unpremeditated way, he makes faces, shouts "no" when I offer something (a slice of bread at table, say, or something I know he likes), bangs his fist on the table in frustration, only to come back and apologize half an hour later, telling me that I had been "too nice" to him, and suggesting that I should be aware that this makes him angry and makes him suffer. What is it that he thinks I might be expecting from him when he gets so angry? Similarly, he also dislikes being treated like a child, pampered and so forth (at least by his parents, for whom—as he well knows—he is no longer a baby, although in the depth of his heart, he still is). He does not want to be loved, and yet . . . He wants either indifference or earnest communication, like that between grownups who don't know each other very well; he loves a joke—although his literal-mindedness prevents him from appreciating more subtle forms of humor or irony—possibly because jokes presuppose a form of distancing, a certain coldness, perhaps even a kind of cruelty, which may be merely symbolic, or rather not, because in fact absurdity is rarely cruel.

As for the creation of personae, or character-masks, I cannot fail to remember Kim, the fictional character invoked by Matthew when he was little, and to whom he attributed all the silly things he did, all his blunders or mistakes, to avoid punishment—he feared being scolded as much as he feared being loved. But this mask of an absent "other," as I understood it at the time, seemed to have a purely pragmatic purpose, namely to deflect possible reproaches or reprimands; it didn't cross my mind that it may have been the sign of a much deeper insecurity. At any rate, that was only a passing phase in Matthew's life. In his own way, as he grew up—and, of course, completely unaware of it—he turned the famous maxim of prudence used by Descartes, "Larvatus prodeo" ("I go forth with a mask"), on its head, replacing it with an implied "Without a mask, I go forth." I am as I am and have nothing to hide. I cannot even begin to imagine how I could hide. I am an open book and I smile. And when I am hurt for whatever reason I get angry, but never hide my anger.

❋

Prompted by a suggestion made by Uta Frith in her book *Autism: Explaining the Enigma* (1989), I borrowed from Classic Film and Music a video of François Truffaut's film *L'enfant sauvage,* 1969 (The Wild Child). I watched it with Uca last night. We were both touched. Of all Truffaut's films about children that I have seen, it is perhaps the most troubling—a haunting masterpiece. After watching it, I immediately reread the chapter devoted by Frith to the wild boy of Aveyron, the feral child whom she considers the first documented case of autism, although the diagnosis is retrospective (the available documents date back two hundred years) and hence speculative. The abandoned child survived as if by miracle in the forest of Aveyron for at least two years, during which he was briefly spotted several times by peasants in the area. He fled from people like a frightened animal. When he was captured, in 1798, he appeared to be around twelve years of age; he was naked and his skin was covered with bloody scratches. A deeply embedded scar on his neck suggested that his parents, or those who had abandoned him, had tried to kill him and had probably left him for dead. But why had they abandoned him when he must have been nine or ten years old? Possibly because he seemed abnormal, and perhaps cried and shouted for no reason (as some autistics do), possibly because he was unable to learn how to speak and could not understand and communicate. When he was caught, the wild child was indeed completely inarticulate, asocial, and, like a forest creature, afraid of people. He was taken to Paris and placed in an institution for deaf-mutes. There the mystery that surrounded him, his unusual story, awakened the scientific and human interest of Dr. E. M. Itard (played in the film by Truffaut himself), who took the boy under his protection into his own home and tried to educate him. With the help of Mme Guérin, Itard invented a series of ingenious procedures to teach the boy—whom he named Victor—to articulate at least a few basic words and recognize the letters of the alphabet. These attempts had only limited success, although Victor made considerable progress in other respects, becoming less fearful of people and more positive in his behavior. Itard wrote a book, *De l'éducation d'un homme sauvage* (1801), the basis for Truffaut's film, in which he follows the boy's life almost up to the moment when Itard abandoned his pedagogical project, although the boy lived on under Mme Guérin's care to be forty-eight.

One of the most arresting scenes in the film is the one in which Mme Guérin and Itard attempt to make Victor utter one word, namely the word *lait*, given that the boy was very fond of milk. (Possible psychoanalytical speculations here: the search for the mother's milk, for the lost paradise of a suckling infant, etc.). The boy's teachers give him an empty mug and then, pointing toward a jug full of milk, repeatedly say "lait." Increasingly impatient, the boy starts shaking his empty mug, making demands with gestures and with imploring looks toward the two, but never uttering the word. Itard finally takes pity on him and asks his collaborator to pour milk into the boy's mug. With a grateful expression and a shrill, strident voice, Victor exclaims ecstatically: "Lait!"—the first articulate syllable he has ever produced in his life—after which he gulps his milk down. Itard's comment on this is interesting: the boy refused to use articulate language to communicate a request, a wish; but he used it—albeit one single, isolated word—to express satisfaction, pleasure, delight, perhaps gratitude. Unable or unwilling to use speech to communicate a wish, the boy could, however, use letters for this purpose, carved wooden letters made especially for teaching him the alphabet; for instance, before being taken on a visit to neighbors, he rushes back to the house, chooses the four letters for the word "lait," puts them in his pocket and then takes them out proudly and displays them in correct order on the table in the neighbors' house. I have read that, in severe cases of autism, typewriters and computers are used as written communication to replace speech.

Truffaut's film, a faithful if, of course, selective reading of Itard's memoir, is a delicately poetic meditation on childhood, on language and the absence of language, on silence . . . Throughout his career as a film director, Truffaut was fascinated by childhood and children and, as such, could not fail to be interested in the enigma of language acquisition—which is the same as the enigma of socialization. Or of failed socialization, in this particular case.

❊

Finished reading *Autism: Explaining the Enigma* by Uta Frith, a British researcher who espouses the so-called theory of mind in cognitive psychology: this is the mentalist perspective, radically different from that of behavioral psychology, which reduces psychological processes to a stimulus-response relationship, ultimately no different from Pavlov's theory of conditioned reflexes based on his experiments with dogs; it is also different from branches of depth psychology such as psychoanalysis, which posits the hypothesis of unconscious traumas and inner drives or impulses. Put simply, the theory of mind is a theory (some prefer calling it a schema) about the interpretive framework that forms naturally in an individual's mind in childhood, a basis from which to attribute desires, intentions, beliefs, and opinions to another individual with whom the child engages in a dialogue or interacts socially. I was not aware of the existence of this new school of thought in psychology and was, therefore, fascinated by everything I learned, and surprised to see that many observations of detail intersected with my own interest in the psychology of reading. For the theory of mind is basically about reading too, in a very broad sense, namely the reading of another's thoughts based on the processing of a multitude of signs (ranging from facial expressions to the sound of the voice, from looks and gestures to other contextual elements), voluntary and involuntary signs that accompany the verbal message proper. (Searching in the university's electronic catalogue for works by the same author, I found that she had indeed written about the psychology of reading and writing, from the perspective of educational psychology. Another interesting work I found in my searches was Henry M. Wellman's *The Child's Theory of Mind,* which I decided to check out.)

Autism, with its triad of dysfunctions (in the areas of communication, socialization, and imagination) is caused, according to Uta Frith, by difficulties in processing verbal and nonverbal information, difficulties that affect a central function of the mind, the one responsible for creating coherence. An autistic person's mind is essentially fragmented because it is incapable of establishing broader coherent configurations, especially regarding information of a social nature coming from the environment. (It is, however, important to note here that this malfunction does not affect the capacity for establishing local coherences and for processing acontextual information; neither does it affect the logical functions of the mind.)

The key to the enigma of autism, according to Frith, is a dysfunction of the capacity for mentally representing—for guessing or "reading"—the mental states of other people. In other words, an autistic child cannot intuit or imagine what goes on in the minds of others (parents, caregivers, classmates, potential playmates). He cannot read social signals: he is like an illiterate person who cannot read the name on the street sign, a street he keeps looking for in vain. He is lost. But while an illiterate person can read social signals (that is, can interpret correctly the semiotic of gestures, faces, clothes, voice tones, and is, therefore, "normal"), an autistic person, although well educated and perfectly able to read the letters, is a rigid literalist—both in the restricted and in the broader sense of the term. It is only with great difficulty and after many explanations that an autistic can understand (most often imperfectly) irony, metaphor, or symbolic analogy. Individuals with autism do not realize, for instance, at what point their words become boring, inappropriate, or meaningless from the listener's point of view. Similarly, they cannot grasp the wider meaning of what they are being told, the allusions, the implications; they have no intuition of what is expected of them, of what they should be doing to please others, or of what opinion others might have of them. Frith calls this the opposite of the mistake made by the roulette player.

The roulette player's mistake is that, as he enters the realm of pure chance, he fails to grasp the perfectly valid principle that in that universe "everything is possible." When considering whether to bet on black or red, he may mistakenly "adopt a theory from which he predicts whether red will turn up next. The gambler is captured by the erroneous belief that there are patterns in chance events and that he can outwit chance. This is a type of gambler's fallacy. Beliefs in patterns and meaning are justified, however, in many situations. These include social relationships and intentional communication. In these situations the gambler's fallacy is not a fallacy. It almost always works!" (p. 179). If the drive toward coherence doesn't make any sense in games of chance, it does, and is even necessary, in the world of human communication, in which one can gamble intelligently and learn from one's mistakes. But for the autistic mind, the patterns of thought and behavior that are to be assembled and understood, in spite of the risk of error, are instead perceived as a collection of disjointed, haphazard, meaningless events. Uta Frith writes that humans "have the possibility of sharing in a wide, wild inner world of relationships and meanings where constant gambles are being taken, and won, and lost. Autistic children, impervious as they are to such gambles, cannot fully participate in such a world. It may fascinate them, or terrify them, but it will not readily admit them as players."

The so-called Sally–Anne or false belief test, administered to children aged three and four, is interesting in this respect. The tested subject is told that a little girl in the group, Sally, has hidden something away, and then the girl leaves the scene. The subject remains at the scene (a room, for example) and witnesses how Anne, another child, moves the object from its initial hiding place to somewhere else (from under an armchair, for instance, to a place behind a curtain). Sally comes back, unaware of what has happened in the meantime. The subject is then asked: where will Sally look for the item? An autistic subject will indicate the place where the item actually is, where Anne moved it, behind the curtain, while a "normal" subject will indicate the place where Sally knows that she hid the object initially, under the armchair (obviously, having left the scene, Sally is unaware that there has been a change). Not all autistic children make that mistake, but most of them will indicate the place where the object really is, not realizing that, of course, Sally will look for it in the place where she knows she hid it. In other words, autistic children cannot imagine themselves in the cognitive position of Sally, who has no idea that the object has been moved behind the curtain.

Undoubtedly, autistic children make attempts to join the social game (I remember how, around the age of six, Matthew wanted to play soccer with other children of his age and rushed toward the ball, kicking it as hard as he could, but in random directions; after a while, players stopped picking him for their team). I would not say that autistic people do not try to guess other people's intentions, but their guesswork is arbitrary; they simply lack a sense of what is likely or unlikely. I agree with Frith that their predictions are based on the principle of chance (anything is possible) or, as in the Sally–Anne test, on what they know to be true, on what they have seen with their own eyes, without taking into consideration the other's likely opinion. But the mistakes made in the social world on the principle of "anything is possible" are too big and too unsystematic for anything to be learned from them. One can only learn from small mistakes.

What persons with autism lack—to formulate Frith's theory in terms that are more familiar to me—is an intuitive referential framework. This is why, as I found out a long time ago, Matthew acquired easily the mechanics of reading—the matching of letters and sounds and pronunciation (which is not easy in English), but has difficulties reading a narrative, a piece of fiction, because he cannot easily play make-believe (or "as if") games as he reads and, therefore, he cannot guess what comes next and become engrossed in the logic of curiosity and suspense, of finding out whether his guess was right or wrong. Autism is, as Frith says, a subtle but tragic deprivation. It is, to quote her again, a handicap "more similar to blindness or deafness than to, say, shyness" (p. 183), but much less evident or immediately observable. Although the deficiency cannot be corrected, or perhaps precisely because it cannot, it is important that parents and educators be aware of it ("Imagine trying to bring up a blind child without realizing that it is blind"; while this would be an impossibility, it is not so in the case of autism, which may be defined as mental blindness, often partial).

Having read this remarkable book, I would make a few observations on Matthew's specific case, observations that I may develop in the future. I noticed a long time ago that Matthew does not tell lies and does not see why anybody else would lie. What is interesting to me—for he knows perfectly well what it means to lie, and that lying is not good—is the fact that lying makes him angry. For instance, whenever we want to excuse his absence from school—like the other day, when Julian, coming from Chicago to see Matthew, stayed at our house—and we tell the school secretary on the phone that Matthew is ill in order to avoid convoluted explanations, Matthew invariably admonishes us angrily: "But that is a lie!" For him, it is clear that one simply should not lie. Innocent or white lies are as bad as any other. A world in which lies are told, a world of cheating, hypocrisy, dissimulation, is a bad, unintelligible world. In a sense, autistics are pure logicians (I reiterate here my reference to Swift's wise horses in *Gulliver's Travels*): for them, communication can only be about what is to the point, about what actually exists. I realize that Matthew's hatred of lying reflects, in a way, the huge difficulties he has with the various forms of lying that are so important in, and sometimes indispensable to, our all-too-human communication.

I do not agree with Frith when she says that the otherworldliness often associated with autism is a mere myth. For me at least, autistic people are fundamentally, radically, and I would even say theologically innocent. Hypocrisy, deceit, affectation, dissimulation, sanctimoniousness, sycophancy, cheating, false representations, con tricks, and all the other forms of corruption related to lying are alien to them. Their innocence is a tragedy, but this does not make it any less innocent. Autistic people lack suspicion. Unfortunately, suspicion is a path to knowledge. Trust is not.

※

How shall I characterize Matthew's attitude to money, now that he is a grown boy? Sometimes he behaves like a stingy man, irrationally stingy, and yet I know that he is not at all tight-fisted. In situations like these, I tell him: "Matthew, don't be so stingy, it's not nice." He smiles without answering. At Kroger's, where the three of us go shopping for food, he is angry when I overspend on what to him are useless items, such as mineral water. Naturally, he does not mind buying drinks he likes, such as Coca-Cola and other soft drinks. We are hardly out of the grocer's when he wants to go to a video games arcade and asks me for money. Is five dollars enough? "Come on, make it twenty!" I give him a twenty-dollar bill, but he rejects it: it is too much, five will be enough. Sometimes he wants to spend from his own savings. At other times, he asks me how much money I've got in my account. Any figure seems to satisfy him: one hundred dollars, one thousand, ten thousand. He likes figures, but when it comes to money, he cannot tell the difference. Sometimes, out of the blue, he asks me to deposit one hundred dollars in his account—or two hundred dollars, or better two thousand. I say yes, but in no time he forgets, and never checks whether the deposit was made or not. A few weeks later, he again suggests all of a sudden: "Could you make a deposit of two hundred dollars into my account?" (Often he suggests thousands.) And then, of course, he forgets all about it, he simply does not seem to care. All these demands, figures, brief chats about money seem unconnected events; they pass without a trace and are not part of broader patterns.

Upon careful consideration, the truth is that Matthew does not have a coherent attitude toward money. Sometimes he can be disinterested and overly generous, at other times he makes all sorts of petty calculations. Occasionally, he appears to have an obsession with money: he has already started to deposit money from his small income into a pension account.

When Uca and I go shopping, we have to hide things away from him when we return home, for fear of his reproach: "You've been spending again!" Yet many times he seems unconcerned. Does he have any concept of what money really is? He probably has more than one, all partial, fragmented, fluctuating, and dictated by changing, isolated, and unconnected circumstances. What he lacks in this area is what Frith calls "a drive toward central coherence." His worries seem to have to do with the future—an abstract but nevertheless threatening future.

❋

With Asperger's observations on "the autistic personality" as a starting point, Uta Frith deals extensively with possible cultural representations of autism in history. Her examples, although highly speculative, are not without interest: for instance, there is the case of Brother Juniper, a disciple of Saint Francis of Assisi, mentioned in the *Fioretti* (Little Flowers), who amazed everyone by the charming literalness of his mind; or the case of the holy fools of old Russia, which "is not only the province of scholars, but has filtered into general knowledge, not least because of Dostoevsky's novel *The Idiot*" (p. 37). On a different level altogether, Frith suggests, the character of Sherlock Holmes could be regarded as illustrating the detached, otherworldly dimension of the autistic intelligence. Here I have difficulties agreeing, although, admittedly, she makes it clear that such images do not reflect the reality, but only the myths about autism. (Sherlock Holmes was a master of "abduction," whereas Matthew is totally incompetent in this area.) I find it even harder to admit that Sleeping Beauty, in her glass coffin, might embody the paradox of "death-like sleep or rather life-like death" (p. 36) and that she could thus symbolize the great physical attractiveness and simultaneous inaccessibility of the autistic child. Frith, like many other researchers, seems to be somehow in love with her subject and as a consequence may be tempted to discover, in the area of cultural history, examples that sometimes look rather far-fetched. Could she be the mother of an autistic child? But I must confess that I myself am not foreign to such temptations.

Modern metaphors for autism such as the "intelligent" computer program, the robot, or the science fiction extraterrestrial seem more apt and closer to Asperger's definition of the autistic personality as an "extreme variant of male intelligence." In this respect, I found Frith's discussion of a computer program called Eliza most enlightening. Conceived by J. Weizenbaum as a tool for analyzing language and reasoning, this program "creates the illusion of perfectly understanding the minds of its partners" (p. 48). The computer's answers to questions posed by humans are always appropriate, encouraging, comforting, or optimistic, according to the situation. Quoting a fragment of a conversation between Eliza and a person complaining of depression, Frith observes, "the conversation becomes gradually more like a psychotherapy session. In this type of dialogue, in which the depressed person thinks 'Eliza' is a therapist, 'Eliza' would be comparable to an autistic person talking fluently and saying the things that are expected in that particular situation, but without empathy." (I believe she is wrong on this point; Matthew, at least, is compassionate—or does he merely give this impression to others?) Frith comments as follows: "As conversation partners or therapists of autistic children we could not help but attribute intentions, even if they themselves did not, and even if the attributions were quite unjustified. It seems to me that psychotherapists who work with autistic children and interpret symbolically what these children do or say would do well to check on this possibility [i.e., that they are like Eliza]" (p. 49).

I am wondering, however: would it be so bad to attribute intentions to such patients if treatment proved efficient? And in any case, it seems to me that treating a human being as a machine is a bigger error than projecting symbolic intentions and reactions upon situations in which the human being in question takes things in a purely literal way. A machine has no understanding whatsoever (and one should include misunderstanding here), whether of a literal or symbolic kind, for understanding presupposes life. In autistic people, literal understanding is a process of life. In their case, the absence of symbolic understanding is a deficiency in a living organism. Likewise disability in deaf or blind people. Whereas a computer program is and will always remain inanimate.

The issue here, as I see it—as the father of a son with autism or Asperger's syndrome or, in other words, as someone who willy-nilly must play the role of therapist/interpreter—the real issue is not looking for symbols where there are none, but trying to understand a human being who is not, whatever might be said, a computer. Is it really true that autistic individuals—even profoundly autistic individuals—lack intentions? I would say that their intentions are sometimes very difficult to grasp, that they do not correspond to our expectations, but that after a while, after a prolonged familiarization, at least some of these intentions can be guessed. And I also believe that we can learn to suspend our judgment and to produce approximate but generous interpretations, adaptable to many situations, no matter how bafflingly complex, or for that matter bafflingly simple, they are.

The computer program metaphor encapsulates a few, but only a few, of the characteristics of the autistic mind (the inflexible literalness, the inability to read social signs) and at the same time makes us aware of the way in which we naturally tend to treat verbal messages, even when they are produced by machines: by attributing intentions, by anthropomorphizing, by projecting our symbolic imagination onto them. I cannot see any harm in treating a machine (and least of all a talking machine) as though it were endowed with human attributes. But the reverse is not true. It is harmful to treat, and even to think of, humans as machines. Could this be the result of the scientific attitude prevalent nowadays? We should always apply Terence's adage: "Nothing human is alien to me." And autistic people are human, too.

*

Matthew bought me a present for my birthday: I found it this morning on the breakfast-room table, placed on the side where I usually take my tea. On top of the nicely wrapped package was a postcard with a mountainous landscape, on which he wrote a few words in his tortured hand. He was present as I opened the package and read his birthday wishes out loud, and I thanked him. He was standing silently, expressionless, aloof. "I want to read the paper," he said, without addressing me in particular. Was it that he felt self-conscious? Or was I attributing to him an emotion that he did not feel? For a moment, I felt like going up to him to thank him once more and give him a hug. But no, he does not like physical contact of any kind, and he detests even from a distance the scent of the eau-de-cologne that I use in the morning as an aftershave. Today, I did not dab my face with it, anticipating exactly this situation, but in any case what would be the point of subjecting him to an affective ritual that disgusts him? So I let him read his sports page in peace. The mere thought of buying me a present and writing a best wishes card was his way of showing affection. He cares for me simply, purely, discreetly, without any need for external recognition on my part.

*

I think that, in spite of the terrible obstacles created in his life by autism, Matthew has achieved a certain inner balance. He is happy in high school— not so much with the results, which he cannot measure and about which he does not really care, because he lacks a competitive approach—but with the fact that he is doing his best (helped with his math by Alexandru Baltag, the "genius" son of my old friend Cezar, and in other disciplines by us) and is coping with all the other demands and requirements of school. I think this makes him feel good about himself. He continues to enjoy school as much as he did in the early years, he likes his teachers, and they are especially sympathetic and kind to him. He has made no friends at · school, but this does not seem to bother him. He appears to have given up the intense desire he had in his younger years for making friends among his schoolmates. Given that he keeps to himself as much as possible, he no longer feels rejected by others, or excluded from their activities and discussions, and therefore he no longer suffers. The other students extend the occasional benevolent gesture, a smile or even a purely conventional question, "How are you doing, M?" which only presupposes the stock answer, "I'm good." They do not really engage with him, but he has come to look upon this avoidance as a natural fact about which he has no reason to complain. He has his moments of pride—when teachers praise him in class, but not when we praise him at home, which leaves him indifferent or even irritates him. What impresses and touches me is to discover in him a number of rare and beautiful character traits: he has a happy nature, in spite of the tragedy that has befallen him; he is at peace with himself; he is not envious or vengeful; he feels no guilt and therefore does not accuse himself or anyone else (I would say that he does not have a concept of guilt, but this does not exclude moments of embarrassment or regret when he makes a mistake or accidentally upsets someone); he has no inferiority or superiority complex.

*

I remember having referred in the past to Matthew's extraordinary auditory sensitivity, especially with regard to tonalities and inflections of the human voice. A touch of spontaneous affection in my voice makes him nervous, and he pretends not to hear, or refuses to answer. But most of all, he is affected by the slightest tone of annoyance or anger, which he can sense even when the anger is otherwise well-contained. Last night around seven, as we were all three having our evening meal, the phone rang and he answered. He then passed the receiver on to me. I realized in a second from the distorted pronunciation of my name—which is impossible to pronounce in English, except by people who try hard because they know me—that it is a cold call, one of those promotional offers for vacuum cleaners or something. The numbers of such cold calls around supper time has increased, and I am extremely irritated by them. "We're not interested," I said, with a tone of voice in which Matthew sensed the nuance of contained anger. He became angry in his turn, but hardly in a contained way. He shouted in revolt, banging his fist on the table and reprimanding me, with a hostile look: "You should've been more polite." I tried in vain to explain to him that these commercial calls—using, it is true, the services of pitiable, poorly paid workers—are in fact brutal invasions of privacy, and so on. He did not understand, and kept repeating: "You should've been more polite." In principle, of course, he was right. Only later did I remember his sensitivity to vocal tones and realize that what he wanted to tell me, but, frustratingly, failed to do, was: "You shouldn't have raised your voice. You know I find it disturbing, frightening, overwhelming." Even during the petty domestic disputes that Uca and I inevitably have (which hardly reach the decibels of their Italian equivalent), Matthew is overcome, as if by some terrifying apocalyptic roars: he covers his ears and howls without stop until Uca and I cease arguing and fall silent. However, the noises he hears on TV, the gunshots, the deafening explosions, the desperate screaming and all that do not seem to bother him. I wonder why. I think it may be because for him the distinction between fiction (whatever comes from the television, images, noises) and reality is radical, as I noticed some time ago; fiction is comforting, while reality—messy, overly complex and unpredictable reality—is what frightens and disturbs him. The slightest trace of anger in my voice is a threat, while violent fighting on the TV screen seems to have a calming effect: it is just a film, fiction, it has no connection with reality. The fact is that he enjoys children's programs shown on Nickelodeon or the Disney Channel, or sitcoms such as the Jeffersons, and cartoons, noisy though they are, more than he enjoys noisy movies per se. At the same time, he is fascinated with wrestling shows, the noisiest of all.

❋

The only good period during the whole of yesterday was late in the afternoon, when I suggested having a game of chess with him; to my surprise, he accepted. He enjoys chess, although he does not play brilliantly—more precisely, he plays unevenly, sometimes very well, sometimes badly. Sometimes he plays chess on the computer against an imaginary opponent. This essentially silent, wordless, and at the same time non-symbolic, abstract game seems to help him focus and distracts him from the painful complexities of daily life, even if only in the ritualized, repetitive forms such complexities take in domestic life. We play two games: one I win, the second I let him win, and he is happy. He is happy because he lost once, and then won once. We are even, nobody has lost, nobody has won.

❋

Last weekend, Julian, Matthew's best friend (with the exception of Phil Wheeler, who, in fact, is more of a mentor to him), stayed in Bloomington for three days. His Mexican-born mother, Nelda, has friends in the department of Spanish here and visits them quite often, especially as she is doing a Ph.D. thesis under the supervision of Frances Wyres and comes for tutorials with her. Two years ago Julian moved with his parents to Chicago, his father having been offered the chair of composition and musical theory at the University of Chicago. Matthew was unspeakably sad; for weeks on end he was in a sort of undeclared mourning. These days he always looks forward to Julian's visits here with great joy—they are an anticipated pleasure, a bright point in a future usually without promise, or with indistinct, barely understood promises.

Julian is about two years Matthew's junior (he is fourteen, Matthew will be sixteen in August) and is suspected of being a high-functioning autistic. But, apart from his rather inexpressive and unfocused gaze, and his occasional avoidance of eye contact, you wouldn't say so. He is a tall, slim, graceful, attractive teenager, moving with an athlete's precision and flexibility. When I once took them both to the university's main gym to practice basketball—it was vacation time and the gym was almost empty—the contrast between Julian's agility and Matthew's awkwardness was striking. In addition, Julian makes an effort both to conform to prevailing fashions among boys of his age, and to stand out, as conventionally unconventional teenagers do here. His clothes are peculiar, at least to me: a worn-out military jacket, jeans trendily torn at the knees, a bicycle chain around his neck, sometimes an even thicker chain with a padlock, hair dyed in garish colors and sprayed into a Mohawk crest. (I once asked him how he managed to do his hair, and he said he didn't do it himself, he went to the hairdresser's.) If I didn't know him, such an apparition would scare me or at least give me the sort of uncomfortable feeling I have on my way to the university when I cross paths with a similarly coiffed and adorned student (there aren't many around, but the few who are are tolerated without comment, perhaps even admired in this permissive campus culture; none of them has ever attended my more advanced courses, but I do have a few students with long hair and rings or other shiny metal studs in their ears or noses, some of them highly intelligent).

For Julian, this accoutrement is undoubtedly a defense, a breastplate behind which hides a delicate, probably quite vulnerable soul. As soon as he opens his mouth, it is obvious that he is a polite, shy, and articulate boy, whose rapid verbal flow is somewhat at odds with his rather weak, velvety voice, ranging in tone between piano and pianissimo: it is a pleasant though unnaturally even voice, with few expressive modulations. He can, however, make his voice sound stronger and fuller, he can speak loudly and stridently, and he does so when he plays with Matthew, imitating some famous TV wrestler. They both enjoy professional wrestling programs, probably because all that sound and fury are mimed and the violence on display is fake. Autistic people's appetite for fake violence, which Phil Wheeler shares, is, I think, due to the apparently paradoxical fact that they themselves are naturally gentle and extremely vulnerable: it is not the violence that they find attractive, but its obviously "fictional" nature, which may have a calming effect on them.

✻

The friendship between Matthew and Julian. Up to the ages of sixteen and fourteen, respectively, both Matthew and Julian enjoyed playing, as I have already mentioned, with stuffed toys, teddy bears of various sizes, some huge, or with the two giant Ninja turtles named Leonardo and Michelangelo—each had a whole collection of them—staging games in imitation of the wrestling shows that they both passionately followed on TV. The toys were given the names of well-known wrestlers, and the two puppeteer handlers gave voice to them, showering themselves with hyperbolic praise, using the ritualized formulae they heard being screamed on TV, in the booming voices of those make-believe athletes, with their apparent violence and their life-and-death pseudo-wrestling: "I am the invincible Goldberg," "I'm the blood-thirsty monster," and the like. In the end, they tired of these games and started playing soccer in the courtyard or, even more enthusiastically, a game they called "brick-ball," invented by Matthew, which involved kicking the ball against the exterior brick wall of our chimney according to strict and complex rules elaborated by the two of them. Then they entered another phase, which still continues, in which they talk endlessly—on the telephone when Julian is in Chicago—about sports results, making forecasts about basketball, football, hockey, or baseball, whatever happens to be in season, and commenting on the performance of their favorite teams or of the famous players they admire.

What strikes me when I hear them talk, and especially, after Julian's departure from Bloomington, when I overhear Matthew on the phone with him for hours on end, is their sheer joy of communicating, without really communicating, just being in touch, hearing their own and each other's voice, a subterranean communication that does not depend upon what they actually say, although what they say is not arbitrary. Sports talk is a mere pretext. What matters is that they are on the same wavelength, and the rest is irrelevant: it does not seem to matter at all that they contradict or agree with each other, that they utter enormities or banalities, that they repeat with patient tenacity what the interlocutor rejects with the same patient tenacity. The relation between Matthew and Julian seems to confirm what Donna Williams says about the need felt by autistic individuals to be with other autistics, about their joy of meeting people of the same emotional age and cast of mind. Their transition from stuffed animals and impersonations to sports marked an emotional growth, I would say. This does not mean that they have actually outgrown an earlier age, but simply that they can hover between the two. In fact, even we "normal" people are not always the same: surely we oscillate between inner ages in much the same way, except that our oscillations are wider, having a greater range? I, too, sometimes get lost in infantile and (unmentionable, of course) teenage reveries, I can be paralyzed by a five-year-old's shyness, and I was until recently the prey of anxious self-created juvenile superstitions: I would make myself strictly follow the same daily route, using the same short-cuts, the same number of steps, touching with my shoulder or my hand the same trees in the same spot, and so on—an autistic search for the self? I, too . . . We are all made of superimposed sensibilities, of different modes of thought and mentalities, but we can navigate more easily among them, we can hide them more efficiently, and we are therefore less vulnerable. We have the ability to lie, which autistic people lack. Because—who can deny it?—lying is one of our basic means of socialization; it can often be our protective armor or even our offensive weapon . . .

❀

Two or three days ago, Matthew had finished his homework for the next day, but it was too early for him to go to bed and he did not feel like playing Nintendo on his own. So Uca suggested reading out loud to him. He reads little, as he finds it hard to pass from words to images, or to engage in the back-and-forth mental movements involved in following even the simplest narrative sequences; it's not that he can't, the effort is simply too great. So she chose, almost randomly, but also because they were short, Aesop's fables, in an illustrated edition. She read out a few fables and he reacted with unexpected enthusiasm. What impressed him most was the fact that those short stories about animals each ended with a moral. He invariably agreed with the moral of the tale (wise, pithy maxims find an echo in his innate moral sensibility), and he would stop and repeat each of them, wanting to discuss them further with his mother. As I listened, observed, and reflected, it seemed to me he took some pleasure in (re)discovering the possibility of language having a double meaning, the possibility of allegorical language. His literal mind was surprised and delighted by this clear possibility—much more oblique, indirect, and difficult to grasp in daily language, with its extraordinarily complex and shifting nuances. The next day, cheerfully, he asked me whether I knew Aesop's fables, "The Tortoise and the Hare," "The Lion and the Mouse," etc. He narrated them to me, happy not only that he could reproduce them, but also that they had a moral, which he asked me to guess. He was very happy when my words came close to the original formulation: it was to him a confirmation that the moral of those fables expressed a generic, incontestable truth. Yesterday, I overheard him having a similar chat with Steve Clark, as they finished their algebra homework for the next day. Matthew even told him "The Lion and the Mouse," which Steve could not remember, insisting on the details (how the little mouse had freed the big lion from the net in which he had been caught by gnawing at the thread), and then challenged Steve to formulate the moral in his own words. He was a proud boy, showing off something he knew about to an adult who listened sympathetically.

At over thirty, Steve is a relatively mature graduate student in mathematics (he took his B.S. only last year), a serious, nice, generous young man who cares for Matthew a lot and who, for reasons that remain obscure, is very fond of handicapped kids. Last year, when I first contacted him to ask him to give Matthew private lessons in algebra, he was working part-time at Cristole House, a home for autistic and retarded children in Bloomington. When he gets his certificate as a secondary school teacher in mathematics next year, Steve told us, he wants to go to teach on an Indian reservation in Arizona, a little-sought-after position. A handsome, athletic man, usually sporting a blond stubble, with gentle but piercing eyes, Steve is like a friend to Matthew: if they finish their algebra early, he is happy to play video games or take Matthew to the basketball court in Bryan Park. Matthew would never think of doing these things with me, although I have suggested many times going to the park to kick a ball around or try our strength on the gym equipment. I am his father and fathers are not supposed to do these things (a father, he once explained to me, cannot be a friend: a father is a father!). The occasional chess game is possible, yes, but . . .

*

Phil Wheeler visited, bringing Matthew a video game he had promised him. Matthew was not at home and, as we waited half an hour for him, Uca and I chatted with Phil. I like him a lot. His relationship with Matthew is long-standing and amazingly enduring. In spite of his handicap (which would be almost invisible if he himself did not mention it), Phil is one of the most rigorously logical, reasonable, and disinterested men I have ever known. I can listen with fascination to his endless autobiographical monologues, to the repetitive, sometimes disconnected sequences of his life as an autistic man, and I realize that—at least to him—autism was a revelation, an almost mystical revelation. Today he has outlined to us what I would call his utopian project (in which Matthew plays a central role) of organizing a small, self-contained society of autistic people, within the larger one, not exactly a "state within a state," but something similar. The more able would educate and help the less able, creating a psychological and moral climate of great beauty and purity, in a word, a real autistic utopia. In this society, Matthew would play a major part: that goodness of his, beyond words, would make him a living example, as he had been to Phil himself. To me this sounds crazy, but I carry on listening with absorbed fascination. Amazingly, Phil presents himself as a disciple of M.! His imagined utopia seems built around a cult of Matthew, who remains completely unaware of his key role.

❉

As Phil Wheeler, carried away by his utopian project, was embarking upon one of his autobiographical detours, Matthew returned home. "At school," Phil was saying, "I thought I was the same as the others, but I was treated differently, I had no friends and I was frustrated and angry inside." "Matthew, too," I said, "believes that others are the same as him, don't you?" Calm and serious, Matthew answered firmly: "No. Everybody's different." Perhaps, I told myself, this (philosophically indisputable) opinion is the reason Matthew has eventually come to accept with serenity whatever happens to him in various social circumstances, the reason why he enjoys school, where, like Phil, he doesn't have friends. One semi-exception is Ian Yeager, a sophomore like himself. He occasionally visits: once he and Matthew went to the Auditorium to see *West Side Story,* another time to see *Pippin,* a play shown at the university theater, and once or possibly twice they stayed in, Matthew having suggested at the outset that they play cards, probably in order to avoid having to talk to his super-articulate schoolmate. I once took Matthew in the car to Ian's house, somewhere remote, near a forest. He lives with his divorced mother who, interestingly, works as a nurse in an establishment for handicapped children. "Everybody is different," Matthew repeats. And if everybody is different, Matthew seems to think, it is entirely normal to be different; implicitly, since everybody is different, one must accept difference—even if one doesn't understand it.

And, of course, trying to be like "everybody else" is entirely meaningless, it is in fact an impossibility, an absurdity: for being like "everybody else" means being what you are, that is, different (paradoxically difference ends up as ... identity). At peace with being different, therefore, Matthew is not trying to imitate anybody in real life; in other words, he has no role model. He loves—or rather, used to love—imitation only in games, and games to him are pure fiction, radically cut off from reality. Ultimately, Phil may be right when he deems Matthew to be an exemplary person in his utopia of a parallel autistic world. In that world, Matthew could be a guru, a guru who doesn't realize he is one, and a role model!

*

When we returned from our short European tour (Matthew had stayed behind, under the supervision of Steve Clark, who stayed with him, and Phil Wheeler, who came daily to check on them), Matthew was waiting at the airport, with Steve. He smiled broadly, welcoming us with wide, touchingly gauche movements of his long arms. He rushed toward Uca to embrace her, and hugged her, happily, with his cheek close to hers. Then he turned toward me, with what seemed to me to be a mix of caution, embarrassment, and genuine desire to be nice. Although I am aware of his built-in dislike of touch, I unthinkingly proffered my cheek, on which he felt obliged to place a brief, hurried, very superficial kiss, after which he withdrew quickly, with a forced smile and an amusingly disgusted expression on his face: "You're wearing cologne," he said, apologetically rather than reproachfully. He hates the scent of cologne, no matter how faint; I remembered, indeed, that I had dabbed my face with lavender after shaving that morning in Paris, many hours earlier. But his olfactory disgust passed quickly, effaced by his joy in seeing us again. "I've brought you a few presents from Europe," I said. "Why? You shouldn't have, you really shouldn't have." Apart from occasions like his birthday and Christmas, Matthew dislikes presents. Does he see them as signs of affection, of which he is afraid? Or is it that he purely and simply doesn't want to be troubled in what I call his asceticism, of which he is entirely unaware? Or does he simply want to avoid being surprised when he is not prepared to be surprised? Before Christmas he prepares himself weeks in advance for the coming surprises.

✻

Why should Matthew like poetry—at least some varieties of poetry—more than prose? Recently, he was delighted when Uca read aloud to him a few poems by Edgar Allan Poe: "The Raven," "Annabel Lee," "For Annie." I am listening in as she reads "For Annie," a poem I used to know by heart as an adolescent, but which I have in the meantime forgotten.

> THANK HEAVEN! THE CRISIS—
> THE DANGER IS PAST
> AND THE LINGERING ILLNESS
> IS OVER AT LAST—
> AND THE FEVER CALLED "LIVING"
> IS CONQUERED AT LAST.
>
> SADLY I KNOW
> I AM SHORN OF MY STRENGTH,
> AND NO MUSCLE I MOVE
> AS I LIE AT FULL LENGTH—
> BUT NO MATTER!—I FEEL
> I AM BETTER AT LENGTH.
>
> . . . .
> THE SICKNESS—THE NAUSEA—
> THE PITILESS PAIN—
> HAVE CEASED, WITH THE FEVER
> THAT MADDENED MY BRAIN—
> WITH THE FEVER CALLED "LIVING"
> THAT BURNED IN MY BRAIN . . .

Does Matthew realize that this poem—quite apart from its soothing metronome-like melody, half-dirge, half-lullaby—is about death conquering the "fever called living"? I doubt it.

❊

The other day, as I was about to go out and do some minor shopping at a local store on Elm Heights Street, I realized I didn't have any change; but, as luck would have it, as I was about to leave, I saw some money on the table in the dining room: thirty dollars, a ten-dollar bill and a twenty. I grabbed the ten-dollar bill (which was more than enough for my intended shopping) and that evening, when Uca returned from work, I told her about it. "It was not my money, it was Matthew's, he withdrew it yesterday from his savings account," she explained. (Uca had, indeed, told me how proud Matthew had been the previous day, when he asked her to drop him off at the bank: he went on his own into the building—he asked her to wait for him outside—and some time later came back with his savings book and the two banknotes, happy, almost triumphant.) "By the way, Matthew," I told him, "I took that money as a loan, I'll go to the Credit Union tonight to get some cash and I'll pay you back." "It's not necessary," Matthew replied. In the evening I handed him the ten-dollar bill, but he refused stubbornly to take it. "But it's your money," I insisted, and, because the phone started ringing that very moment, I rushed to pick it up, leaving the note on the table. Matthew ran after me with the note, repeating: "I don't need this money," and as I was on the phone, he stuffed it into my pocket. "Please don't try to return this money to me. I don't need it," he continued.

But why? He saves it, cent by cent, but in fact he cares nothing about it. At times he appears tight-fisted, avaricious, and possibly is so occasionally, when seized by an abstract fear of an equally abstract, gloomy, menacing future, a future of which he can hardly conceive; otherwise, he is generous, careless even, but at the same time extremely responsible and thoughtful. Does he think that he has an incalculable debt toward us? Or simply that whatever he voluntarily gives, or whatever is taken from him without his knowledge, should not be returned? Is it his incomprehensible fear of reciprocity? I have to resign myself: I shall never understand his way of perceiving money.

❋

(1993) Matthew is celebrating his sixteenth birthday two days early (his birthday is actually the day after tomorrow, the first day back at school). It's a splendid Sunday, with early autumn leaves rustling in the old maple tree at the back of the house: some of them have fallen already, as if "burdened with the light." Two weeks ago I was worried that nobody close enough to Matthew's age would be around (Julian was to be in Chicago). It was possible only Phil Wheeler's much younger sons and, of course, Phil himself, would be able to come. Unexpectedly however, Nelda brought Julian back to Bloomington a few days ago. Good news for Matthew: Nelda has accepted a one-year appointment as a graduate instructor in the Spanish department here, and Julian will stay with her and attend the same school as Matthew. Julian's father will spend the year in Italy on sabbatical. Nelda has bought a small house close to campus and Julian will be staying with us for a week or so while his parents are cleaning and unpacking. Uca has also invited Teddy J. to the party—whom Matthew has not seen in a long time. And, finally, Daniel G., who hasn't come over for more than a year, phoned and was happy to come. So Matthew had an unexpectedly pleasant birthday party and was happy. Happy? He is often happy in his unhappy situation, of which he is not even aware. But is he really happy? Because he forgets the past and ignores the future? *Carpe diem* (seize the day) is a wise maxim (in which Solomon's *Ecclesiastes* meets Epicurean Horace), but for Matthew, who cannot do otherwise, it is a tragedy, with occasional spells of happiness.

❋

Most specialists in autism (from Leo Kanner to Bernard Rimland) agree on one point: the crucial shift toward "normality" happens in adolescence. It is then that autistic persons can grasp the difference between themselves and others. And it is also at that stage that they can start building bridges over the chasm separating themselves from others. If they do not succeed, they will remain prisoners of their singularity and solitude (Uta Frith calls it "autistic solitude") for the rest of their lives. No matter how painful the awareness of difference might be, in the opinion of experts, it is the only realistic chance for social integration, however imperfect or limited. In the preface to *Nobody Nowhere,* Dr. Rimland mentioned the case of his own son, a high-functioning autistic who never grasped his condition and who as an adult led a sheltered life—serene, it would appear, but totally unsociable, at home with his parents.

But Matthew refuses to acknowledge this difference (while in Phil Wheeler's life it was a revelation and turning point when he was first diagnosed as having autism): everybody is different, he maintains. We, however, feel that the moment has come to try to explain to him that he is somehow "more different" than others. I talked to Stine Levy, who has started seeing him for one-hour weekly sessions and, as a therapist, has tried to make him understand and accept his handicap, preparing him for as "normal" a social life as possible. At the beginning, she wanted to establish, as precisely as possible, how he feels about himself, how he per- ceives himself at this moment in time. She constructed a comprehensive questionnaire in order to find out how he himself assesses his strengths and weaknesses: what are the areas where he feels most confident and why? How does he feel at school? How is he getting along with his classmates? Has he got any friends? Does he feel lonely? Which are the areas where he feels he has problems or difficulties? His answers, she told us, were over- whelmingly positive; in other words, Matthew is pleased with himself, he is even quite happy and only admits to a few, very few, areas where he realizes he should do better and be more efficient (he is aware, for example, that he is quite slow in completing some of his schoolwork). He seems so serene and laid-back, he seems to have achieved such a beautiful inner peace, that she, Stine, would not want, would not wish (humanly speaking) to trouble him. In a way, I would say, she has become aware of his beautiful nature, within the framework of his undeniable handicap.

She will continue to see him for some time—he enjoys talking to her, listening to her, taking almost as a form of play the various tests she ad- ministers to him, and this cannot harm him; on the contrary, it might even help him in the future. He takes pleasure in going to see Stine; it is a welcome change in the terrible monotony of his life, especially now, during vacation when he has little to do. But as I observe him at home, I wonder: how genuine is this inner peace that so impresses Stine? And if Matthew is so at peace with himself (as he suggests he is when asked by her), how at peace is he in reality? And what can be done to alleviate the profound boredom that seizes him during his spare time, a time he tries to kill—desperately, I would say—by endlessly watching TV and playing video games on his own? And what can be done about the—albeit unconscious—anxieties arising from that empty time, from that void that threatens to engulf him, in which he can do nothing constructive, nothing that builds cumulatively into a project for a future he cannot even conceive? And what can be done about the permanent state of tension he feels in my presence—the father who cannot be a friend, the father who probably appears to him as unforgiving, severe, excessively authoritarian, even when he pretends to be receptive and benevolent? I'm afraid Stine sees quite a different side of him, a more serene, childish—perhaps more authentic—side, which he doesn't show to me and only occasionally to his mother.

＊

It is true, however, that in spite of the difficulties posed by his autism, Matthew has achieved a certain inner peace that works for him. Now, during vacation, he has come up with a few personal strategies to cope with the oppressive burden of his spare time. In the morning, because of his love of numbers and statistics, he browses attentively through the sports pages in the newspaper, and then on a separate sheet of paper lists the upcoming games with his predictions; later in the day he will compare notes with Julian on the phone. Afterward he plays one or two Nintendo games. Then he takes a break: he sits at the large table in the dining room and he plays solitaire, a game at which he has become very adept. Around lunchtime he leaves home and walks, or gets a lift from one of us, to the College Mall, where he has lunch on his own, paying with his own savings, at one of the restaurants there (Long John Silver's is a favorite). After lunch he likes a stroll around the Mall, always ending up at the video games arcade, Aladdin's Castle. Tired after these basically vacuous games (where he sometimes wins ten or even twenty thousand points—which he can use the next day, invariably losing them—plus five or ten dollars to buy tokens), he is ready for Bryan Park, where he is still taking tennis lessons from Georgianne.

On the days when there is no tennis, he manages to sneak into the softball-training group—for young handicapped people—in preparation for the Special Olympics. Interestingly, Matthew makes no distinction between handicapped children or youngsters (blind, paralyzed, lame, or with missing limbs) and "normal" people. All people are different, and the degree of difference does not matter. He is not affected by—he does not even seem to notice—the fact that someone is in a wheelchair, and if he is addressed he will answer and talk to that person in the same simple, gentle, slow, thoughtful way in which he would talk to anyone. His principle "everybody is different" could also be translated as: everybody has to be treated in the same way. He seems content with the way he spends his days and invariably refuses my repeated invitations to join me on my almost daily hikes to Lake Griffy. In broad outline it could be said, as Stine Levy has suggested, that Matthew has reached a fine balance or—within the strict limitations of his handicap—an unlikely, wise and charming, serenity.

✳

Totally unexpectedly, Matthew has developed a new interest and even eagerness for literature—or more precisely, for the time being, for the kind of fiction that Uca is now reading aloud to him. Matthew has discovered—probably through one of Susan Reed's daughters, who is eleven and whom he sees on occasion—a series of books for children and preteens called *The Baby-Sitters Club,* published by Apple Paperbacks. The series is specifically targeted at children around thirteen years of age who might do baby-sitting for their own and other families in exchange for small amounts of money, or simply to help their parents by looking after a younger sibling when they are out. The little "adventures" that can take place in such situations have to do with some prank of the supervised child, some embarrassment from which he or she is saved by the club girls, some unexpected event requiring presence of mind.

Such things excite Matthew's enthusiasm, and I can see why. During the reading, he clearly identifies with one or another of the main characters, who appear in all the volumes of the series (over a hundred so far and still going strong). But he likes the young children in the books the most because, as I have noted over the years, he has a strong, mysterious affinity with young children, based on his emotional age of three or four. This situation has been rendered quite complex, however, by his advancing mental age, which has reached and passed the time when a sense of moral responsibility forms and starts growing. At any rate, it is the first time that I've seen Matthew fully engaged in the make-believe games through which readers of fiction are carried to a different world. Matthew is not attracted to adventure fiction with adult heroes—fights, escapes, shipwrecks, dangerous searches, romantic love, sudden reversals of fortune, and the like—because he almost certainly does not have the heroic or erotic fantasies of "normal" adolescents. I think I'm right in guessing that his fantasies involve him playing roles of responsibility among children who need protection, helping them to get out of unpleasant or dangerous domestic situations, comforting them when they cry, guiding them when they do something wrong. This appears to be the form taken by his heroic fantasies. In common with most autistic people, he seems to lack erotic fantasies—at least for the time being.

For several days now, before going to work at the university art museum, Uca reads one of these short novels to him, for an hour or even longer: this has become a new vacation ritual. They sit together on the blue sofa in the living room, and Uca holds the book open so that he can get a good view of the page: he likes following the text she reads line by line, word by word. He is keen to see the text as he listens. The conversion of letters, words, and sentences into a slow flow of meaningful sounds may appear to him as some minor form of magic. He laughs cheerfully at amusing passages, interrupts the reading occasionally with perplexed questions, and is happy to see the story resume. The story obviously interests him, he anticipates things, is curious about what comes next, tries to guess the

solutions to the various problems the main characters face. He is so engrossed in the plot that when Uca has to answer the phone, for instance,
he is too impatient to wait and continues reading on his own. Once, when
Uca was busy, he read an entire chapter aloud himself. I observed him
discreetly: he was reading with concentrated attention, articulating each
word quietly, correcting his pronunciation when necessary, in order to
connect the words on the page in meaningful, natural-sounding sentences
and idiomatic expressions. I was pleasantly surprised to hear him adapt
his voice, when dialogues came up, making it sound like a girl, a boy, or a
child, for each of the different characters.

                                          ✳

Uca has read what I've written so far in this diary about Matthew, and
although she agrees with many of my observations on individual points,
she differs with me about the portrait as a whole. Too many shadows and
half-shades, a vision too gloomy and pessimistic. Matthew is not—as I
have portrayed him—anxious or bored that often. There is much more
light around him and in his life. My vision may be darker due to my own
difficult, overly cerebral nature, which makes my relationship with him
tenser and more complicated; this, in turn, is reflected in his somewhat ap-
prehensive attitude toward me. Uca's relationship to Matthew is different:
it is warmer, more open, richer in nuances, more natural. This is why, from
her perspective, Matthew seems neither bored nor anxious, nor overly concerned with finding ways to kill time. On the contrary, when he is with
her, he behaves as though he has too many things to do, confronted, as it
were, with an embarrassment of riches. When he finally makes a decision
to do something, he is happy. In her company, he is generally relaxed—far
from being tense, as I see him, he is affectionate and sincere, although like
anyone else he has his bad days and throws an occasional tantrum. But his
customary disposition is much calmer, sunnier, and more benevolent than
what would be gathered from my pages.

But what is the truth of the matter? I believe both images are justified
and true to a point, beyond which the contrasts sharpen because Uca and

I expect different things from him, and he reacts differently in turn. So much in personal relationships depends upon mutual adjustments among expectations, wishes, or intentions, which can either be accommodated or countered, often involuntarily or unconsciously. Moreover, one may ask: what role do mistaken interpretations of the other's unspoken thoughts and the fear of mistaken interpretations play in a relationship? And what of simulation and dissimulation—how important are they for open, genuine, essentially honest communication? Is it not possible, for example, that a so-called white lie may sometimes lead to more authentic communication (including emotional communication) than a rigidly formulated truth? Such matters are complex and delicate enough, but in the case of a teenager with autism, they are infinitely so. Or is it me—complicating things and thus disturbing my relationship with Matthew?

But rather than raise such abstract and ultimately unanswerable questions, perhaps I should use these pages simply to record what happens to Matthew in the humble context of daily life: his actions, his small discoveries, successes, failures. A recent success, for instance, primarily owing to Uca: Matthew read an entire book on his own, from the aforementioned series, and was extremely proud. He started by reading aloud, but halfway through, his mother encouraged him to read silently, as he has seen us doing, and, miraculously, he began doing so (pronouncing the words in his mind; I don't think he is capable yet of purely visual reading). It took him a few hours of intense concentration, and when he finished, around half past nine that evening, he was nearly ecstatic. His face radiated happiness. He wished to share this intense reading experience at once by telling Uca the story in a loud, enthusiastic voice. Because he wanted to repeat the characters' words exactly, he resorted to the book at what seemed to him key moments in the story, modulating his voice, in a kind of naïve dramatic reading. I observed this extraordinary scene in silence.

❋

Last night after supper I went for a walk with my colleague H.M., a specialist in biblical studies, and Matthew remained on his own. When I returned about two hours later, I found him sitting in the same spot, engrossed in reading. He had been reading without interruption, obviously captivated, Uca told me. Being captivated by reading, a psychological phenomenon I explored five years ago in Chicago in connection with my study on reading, was something I had never noted in Matthew either before or after that time, until now; I am glad that he has crossed this threshold, although somewhat belatedly. When he got up from his chair and put his book aside to get a glass of Sprite from the kitchen, he glanced by chance at the clock on the window sill: "It's half past nine already! That's impossible!" he exclaimed in amazement. What a wonderful and pleasant surprise for him: as if (and I am speculating here) time stood still for two hours. This was apparently new to him, although it is the common experience of readers caught up in a story, participating in it so intensely they forget the real world. With the possible exception of some movies, nothing but this absorbed, self-hypnotic reading could produce in him the retrospective illusion of having been outside time, transported to another world. But don't we all read both for the delights of the story line, and for the subtler, less straightforward pleasure of exiting ordinary time, breaking that implacable flow in which, as Matthew remarked suddenly the other day, "one never grows young"? I wonder where he learned the truth (perhaps in his natural science class?) that all living creatures inevitably grow old, that nothing grows young, that time is a never-returning arrow? "One never grows young"—a melancholy thought for someone who might secretly wish he could grow backward, from youth to childhood. But growth, as he has become aware, is irreversible.

Now that he is sixteen, Matthew must be conscious of the gap between his chronological and emotional age. In his own way, he has assimilated the social conventions that prevent an adolescent from behaving like a child. "One never grows young"—I too find that a melancholy observation, although my melancholy differs from his. Unlike him, I have a sense of the future, as shrinking, diminishing with every day, pushing me ever closer to the looming, yet unpredictable moment of my abrupt transition from one to zero, the moment when the infinitesimal collapses into nothingness. "One never grows young," Matthew said, out of the blue, just once, but this banal yet true statement has lodged in my mind. He uttered it free of any context: one of those universal truths to which he seems to have such easy access.

But—to leave the rarefied world of metaphysical considerations about death—the books that Matthew currently enjoys and which he likes to retell to his mother, in spite of his lingering linguistic and sequencing difficulties, are books that, while satisfying his need for imaginative engagement in the world of children, also instill in him a sense of how inappropriate it is to behave childishly when one has outgrown childhood. For example, while recounting one of these stories, he was amused by the fact that a twelve-year-old girl had a poster of Humpty Dumpty on her bedroom wall. "Imagine that!" he said, laughing. "To be twelve and have a Humpty Dumpty poster."

*

Yesterday, Uca and I had a lengthy discussion about Matthew with Stine Levy, who has seen him weekly for the last three months. We all agreed that for the time being he has no need of extensive psychotherapy, which might harm the healthy mental balance he has achieved. "For many autistic people," Stine told us, "achieving a positive self-image like Matthew's would probably be unattainable through psychotherapy. It seems to me a miracle that Matthew has such a positive and proud self-image." The word "miracle" took me completely by surprise: I've always thought of her as a serious professional who weighs her words carefully and avoids awakening unwarranted hope. She certainly did not leave any room for false hope eight years ago when—unlike Dr. E.S. from Indianapolis, who evaded the issue with the phrase "atypical developmental disorder"—she told me straight out, with almost brutal candor, in a conversation I will never forget, that Matthew was autistic. She explained what autism was and stated clearly that it was a "pervasive," incurable condition that remained essentially unchanged for the life of the individual affected and was not limited to early age, as the now discarded term "infantile autism" might suggest. I was shocked, but I respected her for her integrity and honesty. (Of course I reminded her she had misdiagnosed Matthew four years earlier, and she admitted her error. She had grown professionally in the meantime, she added.)

In yesterday's conversation, Stine spelled out in greater detail what she had said to Uca over the phone the week before: that it would be a shame— at least at this stage—to destroy the self-confidence of someone affected by autism, or rather by its less severe variant, Asperger's syndrome, which she believed was what more accurately described Matthew's condition. She insisted on the term Asperger's syndrome and advised us, when we spoke to Matthew about his "difference," to use this term rather than autism. Autism was almost always diagnosed in severe cases in which profound mental retardation and nearly total lack of articulate speech were common. Eight years earlier, when Asperger's article was still unknown to American professionals, she had referred to Matthew's condition as high-functioning autism. If we referred to it simply as autism, Matthew might hear about it on TV or in films, where it is generally presented as a serious handicap, and be disturbed. From what she says, I gather that for an increasing number of people who understand it imperfectly, autism is a stigma. The term seems to have acquired the same negative connotations leprosy once had, or AIDS today. Fortunately, experts—and this is apparent in the new DSM III-R (Diagnostic and Statistical Manual of Mental Disorders, third revised edition)—are now making an increasingly clear distinction between Asperger's syndrome and classic autism. "When I talked to you eight years ago," Stine told me, "I didn't know what I know now. I thought then that I knew everything there was to know about autism, but now that I know more, I realize how little I know."

Our aim, when we arranged for Stine to see Matthew regularly, was to bring him to an awareness of his "difference" (he himself is so naïvely and perhaps philosophically unaware of it). The assumption was that only such awareness, no matter how painful, might make Matthew want to integrate socially, to the extent of his abilities. We have been influenced, we told Stine, by the widespread belief, shared by doctors and their more articulate patients alike, that patients experience a sense of relief and even liberation when they learn of their handicap. In theory this revelation might motivate them to make a special effort to find a social niche in which to lead an active life. We cited the case of Phil Wheeler, Matthew's older friend (with whom Stine was familiar: she first diagnosed him and she occasionally sees and advises him even now), and the case of Donna Williams, described in such dramatic and moving detail in her memoir *Nobody Nowhere*. But, according to Stine, Matthew's case does not really fit in with these. She told us: "Donna Williams experienced true trauma—unspeakable suffering and endless frustrations—before she discovered she had autism. And the same is true of Phil. In such situations it is surely a relief to discover your true condition, because it explains and gives meaning to the otherwise senseless suffering you have experienced. But Matthew's experiences, ever since he was a baby, have been positive. He is self-confident and comfortable with himself. He does not feel socially rejected, or at least he doesn't suffer from it. And this gives him an admirably positive self-image—no matter how inadequate he might appear from someone else's perspective."

She continued: "I asked him, for instance, if he is being bullied by schoolmates. 'Not really,' he answered, 'and if they do, I ignore them.' 'Are there things that make you unhappy or annoy you?' 'Yes, sometimes, but I ignore those, too.' He seems to have developed his own technique for facing difficult situations. How he did it remains a mystery to me. It is simply miraculous. He is capable—and his case is unique in my experience with autistic children—of isolating himself from whatever might disturb his fundamental serenity. And this is what makes him so charming. For he is indeed an attractive and charming boy, and this quality will prove valuable in the future. He is an engaging young man and he likes to know that he is appreciated."

"Did he seem to be aware, or even marginally aware, that he's different?" I asked Stine at some point. "Not at all. I asked him a lot of questions, direct and indirect, about it, and he never gave any indication that he feels set apart. At first, I wanted to see what he thought the purpose of our meetings might be. I offered several suggestions. Perhaps he came to see me to find out more about himself? 'But I know who I am. I know my name and address. I know the grade I'm in at school. I know the school I'm in. What else is there to know?' Like other people with Asperger's syndrome, Matthew is an absolute literalist. He sees the world in black and white, with nothing in between, no gray areas, no nuances, no gradations. Whatever isn't black is white; black is bad and must be ignored—that's his implicit way of reasoning."

Stine's observations about Matthew's naïve, Manichean, black-and-white worldview suddenly opened my eyes about some opinions to which he is obstinately attached and which he repeats in rather disconcerting ways. If, for instance, when he comes home from the cinema, I ask: "What was the movie like?" he replies "Good." "How good?" "Good. All movies are good." "In what way? Did you enjoy it more, or less, than other movies?" "What do you mean, enjoy it more? All movies are good. All movies are equally good." What I now understand is that Matthew meant going to the movies is good in itself, it was an experience he placed in the "white area." He takes my question in generically literal terms and communicates, in equally generic-literal terms, that watching a movie is a "white area" event. And white is white. He is undoubtedly annoyed that I fail to understand this and keep asking the same question, "How was the movie?" when I should already know the answer. The distinctions he makes among the various movies he sees—his value judgments—take a different, nonverbal, form (which shows that after all he is aware of nuances): the movies he enjoys very much he wants to see several times (five, six, seven, even ten times), while those he likes less he doesn't care to see again. When I told Stine the story about the movies, she said she was not at all surprised.

Matthew envisages his future in the same black-and-white terms. Stine told us: "When I asked him what he wanted to do when he graduated from high school, he answered immediately: 'I'll go to university, of course.' 'Which university or universities do you have in mind? Do you have any preferences?' 'Why should I? All universities are the same, aren't they?' Then I asked him to enumerate a few universities he had heard of. 'Indiana, Purdue, Ohio State, Indiana State, Brigham Young . . .'" I wonder why Matthew did not give a longer list; he knows dozens of college basketball teams from the games he watches constantly on television. But it was clear that universities, too, were in the "white area." Along the same lines, Stine told us that in the nonverbal test she gave him, Matthew considered every question he thought particularly difficult with care, then ended up by skipping them, although he knew that he jeopardized his final score by doing this. He did not want to have to guess. She encouraged him to do so—there was always a chance that he might guess correctly—but he refused. "For him it was strictly a question of whether or not he knew the right answer. If he did, fine, if he didn't, that was that, he skipped. Guesswork has no place in his black-and-white world. Either you know with certitude, or you don't. If you have to guess, it means you don't know and, therefore, you are in the 'black' zone, even if you hit upon the right answer." I wanted to tell her—but didn't—that Matthew would have considered guesswork cheating, to which he has a total aversion, along with treachery and lying. He took the test Stine gave him, as he does at school, seriously, with respect for the truth and the duty of being truthful. He could not regard a test as a game. Had it been a game, he would have been more than happy to guess (in games, one must guess). It is perhaps another example of literal-mindedness. The domains are strictly separated.

But does Stine think Matthew has a real chance of going to university? Her answer is cautious. A technical school such as Ivy Tech in Bloomington would be a possibility. She mentioned this to Matthew, but he appeared unenthusiastic, perhaps because Ivy Tech is not a real university, and he cannot conceive of going to anything other than a real university. Another possibility would be the small, private University of Indianapolis, which I had not heard of: one of her patients, a young twenty-year-old, is a student there and seems happy (the university even devised a special program for her). The University of Indianapolis specializes in teaching students with learning difficulties and handicaps alongside ordinary students. The atmosphere would be good for Matthew, Stine told us: "Matthew is an intelligent teenager. I gave him a nonverbal IQ test and his score was above the average for his age. He scored 113, which is consistent with what he scored on the same test at the age of four and a half, when I didn't have the remotest idea he might have autism. [Interestingly, she has kept the results of these tests in Matthew's file.] This means he hasn't lost anything in terms of nonverbal intelligence. Soon I'm going to give him a verbal intelligence test—where his score will certainly be lower—and that will give me a more precise idea of his academic capacities."

"What would you say his present emotional age is? Three, four, more?"
I asked her, obviously influenced by Donna Williams, but also by my own
earlier observations. "That's a difficult question. In certain respects, he
might be three or four emotionally, but the mechanisms he's developed to
block out unpleasant experiences could not have been devised at such an
early age. Defense strategies are normally conceived at a later age—nine,
ten, eleven, or perhaps even twelve years of age—and rarely function as
well as they do in Matthew's case. It's an amazing achievement. When
bullied by other children, four-year-olds are normally defenseless. But I
have to say that 'emotional age' is not a concept we psychologists work
with, because there are no good ways to measure it. With respect to social
age, which is a clearer concept to us, I would place Matthew somewhere
between seven and eight. But intellectually, as his results in algebra indicate, he's at a more advanced level. I'm really curious to see how he scores
in the verbal intelligence test."

I asked Stine about the sexual life of teenagers with Asperger's and
mentioned Matthew's seemingly total lack of erotic interest in girls—or
boys. His wrestling matches with Julian may have had an erotic component; at any rate, they occasionally discussed what it meant to be gay. She
told us that based on her experience teenagers affected by the syndrome
fall into two clear categories: some have a strong sexual drive (they may
masturbate four or five times daily, which provides one of their few pleasant experiences in an otherwise miserably monotonous and horizonless
life, full of anxiety and fury), while those in the second category have a
weak or nonexistent sex drive, although not to the point of impotence.
To illustrate the second category—which seems to be Matthew's case, at
least so far—she told us about one of her patients with Asperger's, a highly
successful young man who works in a bank, lives alone in a rented apartment, has a driver's license and a car, and so on. For a while he toyed with
the idea of finding a girlfriend (like most young men, whom he wished to
emulate), but after a good deal of hesitation and deliberation, he gave up the
idea. He's not in the least interested in having sexual relations and prefers
living on his own, without the comfort, but also without the responsibili-
ties, of a relationship. [As I am transcribing these lines, I'm reminded of
Oliver Sacks's essay on the case of Temple Grandin, an autistic woman with

a Ph.D., who became famous for her insightful autobiographical articles and books, such as *Emergence: Labeled Autistic* (1986) and *Thinking in Pictures: And Other Reports from My Life with Autism* (1995). When Oliver Sacks asked her about her views on sexual intimacy, she replied that she had no views at all: "She was celibate. Nor had she ever been dated. She found such interactions completely baffling and too complex to deal with; she was never sure what was being said, or implied, or asked, or expected. (. . .) This was common with autistic people, she said, and one reason why, though they had sexual feelings, they rarely succeeded in dating or having sexual relationships" (*An Anthropologist on Mars*, p. 285).]

"Might Matthew have a private life?" I asked Stine. "The answer is no," she said. "Then he is as he seems to be," I continued, "an open book. He has no 'secrets,' he is a perfectly transparent young man." "Yes," she said at the end of our conversation, "but you must be aware that this adds to his already considerable charm. This charm will be a great asset to him in life. My prognosis for him is good, very good."

❋

Yesterday we went to the reception given by Christina for her summer session students. Among the guests were two visitors from Romania (on Fulbright and Hubert Humphrey grants) and Christian M., who gave up his assistant professorship in Bucharest to become a graduate student in comparative literature here—somewhat tense, with a tendency to avoid eye contact, but with great strength of will; I think he will do well. Matthew behaved very reasonably. He talked to some of the guests—the usual chit-chat among people who have just met, simple questions (Where are you from? What's your subject of study?). As we left, Matthew was jubilant: "That was a very nice party." He copes remarkably well in social situations where communication is predictably superficial, polite, and literal.

"Are you looking forward to the start of the school year?" his mother asked him on the way home. (He returns to school on 24 August, the exact day he turns sixteen.) Matthew seemed slightly surprised and was silent a while, then gave his usual response: "I don't know" ("I don't know" often means "Leave me alone" or "Don't pester me"). His mind was elsewhere, in another frame of reference; perhaps he was still thinking of the pleasant encounters he had just had, his thoughts were far from school, and he was unable to shift his attention and give a focused answer. In Matthew's case, "I don't know" summarizes his difficulties not only in communicating but also in shifting attention. He could simply reply "yes" or "no" but that would not be truthful. He also realizes that a "yes" or "no" calls for further explanations. "I don't know" is his way of cutting off an unwelcome discussion.

※

Over the past few days, I have been reading a number of articles from the collection *Natural Theories of Mind: Evolution, Development, and Simulation in Everyday Mindreading,* edited by Andrew Whiten (1991). This subject has fascinated me ever since I first read Uta Frith's book on autism. Her thesis is that autistic people are by nature incapable of acquiring and using a theory of mind, or do so only with the utmost difficulty. The more I read about this subject, the less convinced I am that a deficit in mind reading as such is the key to the enigma of autism. I find Paul Harris's incisive article "The Work of the Imagination" very persuasive in his nuanced skepticism about this hypothesis. Harris rejects the very existence of a theory of mind in children. Difficulties or relative lack of expertise in reading other people's minds is not the cause of autism but rather one of its possible symptoms. At least as important is another symptom—directly affecting processes of analogy, on which mind reading itself is based—namely, a difficulty in rapidly shifting one's focus of attention, which I have observed many times in Matthew. Because this difficulty also hinders one's ability to divide one's attention between two or more simultaneous events, the autistic child's predictions are often mistaken and he or she begins to expect that such mistakes will be repeated, which may lead to a paralyzing fear of error, social anxiety, and a tendency toward withdrawal.

[When I wrote these lines, I was unaware of the major study of Simon Baron-Cohen, *Mindblindness: An Essay on Autism and Theory of Mind*

(1995). The author attempts to explain the absence of the so-called theory of mind in autistic children by a deficit not so much of attention proper as of "shared attention," which can be observed as early as the age of eighteen months. But what is shared attention? When the mother looks toward an object, the baby tends to direct his or her gaze toward the same object or at least in the same direction, without other prompts. The beam of the baby's attention intersects with the mother's and is directed toward the same object. This would be a first, very early, psychological mechanism, a form of nonverbal dialogue appearing prior to the first elements of language, or at about the same time, and signifies the beginning of a mutual understanding of minds, a spontaneous coordination of attention based solely on gaze. A lack of such coordination, according to Baron-Cohen, is an early symptom of autism. As for the term "mindblindness," which he coined, it appears to me to be an imperfect, if useful, analogy. I would prefer to call it, especially in Asperger's cases, a severe mental shortsightedness (only partially, if at all, correctable by behavioral therapy), which fails to read many, though not all, social signals, and fails to read especially the relations between these signals. In other words, the perception of social cues is fragmentary and the fragments are unrelated. But this may after all amount to a sort of blindness, as Baron-Cohen claims.]

＊ Why am I keeping this diary about M? The answer is simple: because I want to understand him, and I want to understand him because I love him both as my son and as a unique human being. I love him not only because he is innocent and good, an intensely moral being, but also—perhaps primarily—because he is unique. And because I want to help him all I can. But understanding is by no means simple: the equation to be solved includes numerous conflicting attitudes, a combination of (perpetually readjusted) expectations, recurrent hope-against-hope, and constantly renewed attempts at a unified solution. So many puzzles, some of them quite concrete, others of a metaphysical or existential nature, are essentially insoluble. Finally, understanding involves—and this complicates things further—understanding oneself through the other, and the other sometimes bears only an apparent, perhaps misleading and illusory resemblance to oneself. How can one penetrate such illusions? All this, I know, sounds terribly abstract. What do I mean, for instance, by "conflicting attitudes"? On the one hand, there is the spontaneous, instinctive attitude of parental love, protecting, generous, always striving toward empathy and emotional transparency; on the other, there is the fact that such empathy and transparency are impossible to fully achieve, that—in Matthew's particular case, once I became aware of it eight years ago—they can give rise to distorting or falsifying projections. And there is the fact that something obscure resists natural, unmediated understanding—hence, the curiosity, the intellectual desire to find explanations, to clarify the causes of something that appears abnormal, or the desire to understand my son's condition in a "scientific" way, by reading medical literature on similar cases and trying to find out about possible therapies (or at least about marginally effective therapies, if there is no cure).

How can I describe the purely intellectual interest of such readings, doubled as it is by the immense personal anxiety and despair they often produce? All I can do—driven as I am by a parent's love within a tragic situation (my definition of tragedy: an awareness that disaster is inevitable and must be accepted as part of a necessarily broader script)—is to tell myself that the attempt to understand must continue. Must. But what could that necessarily broader script be? I would say that its nature is statistical—what I termed some time ago the genetic or biological lottery. But what of the existential enigma? To put it naïvely: what is the meaning of life? The meaning of suffering? That life is a miracle I do not doubt. But, likewise, I do not doubt that this miracle generates numberless statistical tragedies—as well as the certitude of death. Can life, therefore, be said to be an *absurd* miracle, a miracle without a point? Or is a theological vision preferable, one that turns absurdity into mystery? Such questions may seem silly—of course, they could be given a certain philosophical "dignity" by a more refined mode of expression—but they are also poignantly topical, intense, unavoidable. In any case, this search for understanding—including an understanding of my own anxieties, of my depression, my solitude, and my struggle to suppress such negative feelings in order to help

Matthew—continues unabated. This diary is just a modest, intermittent, insufficient testimony of that search.

❋

Yesterday I heard Matthew on the phone with Julian. They were having one of their usual lengthy conversations. The main topic was the world soccer championship. But at some point, the discussion turned to death. This surely had to do with the shocking news of the Colombian player Andres Escobar, who, playing against the United States, had scored by mistake against his own team, and was killed by furious fans. Matthew was telling Julian in a consoling tone that the soul of someone who dies goes to heaven. Julian must have expressed some doubts, for Matthew emphasized in a firm tone: "I do believe in God." That evening, in his sleep, he had a terrifying seizure, he was thrashing about as if possessed, and I watched him moaning helplessly for what seemed an eternity.

❋

I continue to reflect on what psychologists call everyday mind reading, the ability to read someone else's thoughts spontaneously, instantly, and effortlessly. What an important role this ability plays in ordinary communication! It is a role we take for granted in daily life. But mind reading is only a shorthand way of referring to an infinitely complex process that has as much to do with communication itself as with meta-communication, the latter comprising the facial, gesticulatory, phonetic, and only occasionally verbal, suggestions that, in any given situation, indicate how a message should be taken by the one to whom it is addressed, the framework in which it should be decoded (the metaphor of reading again!) to adequately understand the person who utters it. As I have learned, autism and Asperger's syndrome have more to do with difficulty in decoding meta-communicative signs than with the understanding of the strictly logical content of a speech act. This means that all strictly linguistic conventions, which high-functioning autistics can master, are deeply embedded in other conventions, second-order conventions, which contain the indications for how first-order conventions should be interpreted. The notion of mind reading includes these second-order conventions (minor signals, spontaneously identified referential contexts, suggestions, implicit "stage directions," etc.), but these do not necessarily express the speaker's true intentions (these real intentions could be to cheat, to lie, to hide). Actually, these second-order conventions are as conventional as first-order ones, only less systematic, less formal, less clear, which means they allow for more ambiguity. Even "normal" people sometimes misconstrue them, leading to what Irving Goffman calls "frame break-ups"—for instance taking a humorous threat seriously, feeling insulted by something that was meant as mere teasing, or interpreting *ad litteram* an irony. A communication succeeds only when its temporary, ephemeral, contextual function is properly understood. At this level, people with Asperger's often make mistakes. They are blind or rather partly blind when confronted with meta-communicative allusions or suggestions, which by their very nature are more fluid than purely linguistic conventions. Hence the possibility of deception, which the autistic mind cannot comprehend. I think that even if they could become proficient in mind reading, autistic persons would be literal-minded even on this level: trusting, incapable of lying and of imagining that they could be lied to, they would take what they are told as well as the manner of telling at face value. Their minds seem to be programmed exclusively for truth. This is a major handicap.

*

It has been said that autistic people show no personal initiative, lack motivation and self-motivation, and live in a state of inner inertia. Matthew seems to belie such generalizations. He often has personal initiatives and is capable of making efforts to achieve them. His problem is that such initiatives—although occasionally passionate—are short-lived and do not connect with others, do not combine to form patterns. Yesterday, for instance, he wanted to learn a certain song from a movie he loves, *A League of Their Own*. He began by writing the lyrics down word by word as he watched the video recording, playing the soundtrack over and over. He spent two intense hours this way, stopping the tape repeatedly to catch each word and write it down in his childish, slow hand. When he was not sure of a spelling, he came to ask me, but without telling me what he was doing and why; "How do you spell this or that word?" Absorbed in my own reading, I thought for a while that he was writing to Julian. I finally saw that the words he was asking about (such as "chaperone") came from the film *A League of Their Own,* which he had tape-recorded and watched several times, "forcing" us to watch as well. Maybe he was writing Julian about the film. . . . But no, what he wanted was to learn the lyrics of one of the songs from the movie by heart. This may seem a simple thing, but I now know that such simple things, which we take for granted, involve almost miraculously complex mental operations, even when they are essentially mechanical, such as identifying the words in a continuous flow of music and text, which when recorded can be stopped and started. And there is the element of self-motivation prompting one to act, that nexus of pleasure and "work for pleasure" without which the accomplishment of any initiative would be impossible. Later, he proudly sang the song for us, pronouncing each word clearly, but in a continuous high falsetto since, unfortunately, he totally lacks an ear for music.

He had done this before. Whenever he came across a song he liked, he wanted to copy it out, word by word, in his own handwriting. The other day I found, on a large piece of paper—the back of an old, unused desk calendar—the text of another song he had written down, "Lean on me": "Sometimes in our lives/We all have pains/We all have sorrows/But if we are wise/We know that there's/Always tomorrow./Lean on me when you're not strong,/Then I'll be your friend, I'll help you carry on/For it won't be long till I'm gonna need/Somebody to lean on." Together in suffering, you today, me tomorrow. But, as I said, these words do not connect for him, do not lead anywhere, and their echoes are quickly forgotten.

✻

Just back from the airport, where I drove Uca and Matthew en route to Washington, D.C., and then to the National Institutes of Health where Matthew will be admitted to the Epilepsy Section for clinical tests—these may take a week or more. He will be hooked up to an encephalograph all the time and undergo a host of other tests. Uca will be with him, sharing his room at the clinic. On Friday I will be visiting them for three days. In his muted way, Matthew was looking forward to the hospitalization in the hope that some remedy might be found to his increasingly frequent and severe seizures. Aside from them, but perhaps in connection with them, he has had a weight loss of about forty pounds over the last few months (from 190 to 150). At the airport, when we parted, he kissed me lightly on both cheeks (overcoming his usual reluctance, perhaps because he himself initiated the move). He looked at me: there was a sadness in his beautiful eyes, but also, I believe, a glimmer of hope and expectancy. Silently, without any outward gestures, he was excited by the trip.

*

Why did Matthew enjoy (he said: "It was great!") the ten-day stay at NIH? (For Uca, who spent all this time with him in the clinical building, it must have been rather an ordeal, but she underwent it resignedly, calmly, with a courageous stoicism.) It must have been the social context that made the difference for Matthew. Nurses came and went all the time, smiling, asking simple questions, showing kindness and concern. In other words, he was at the center of attention of a host of people, and this outweighed some painful episodes (his terrible headache and backache after the lumbar puncture, the need to lie motionless for two or three days afterward, the drawing of blood for different tests, the skin graft for the DNA, among others). His state of quasi-euphoria could have derived from the fact that patients in a hospital are somehow infantilized, and this made him feel securely installed, without any challenges, in his deep childish self. At any rate he won the reputation of an ideal patient at the NIH, and the nurses loved him. When he was dismissed, one of the nurses, Jeni, said she was sorry he was leaving and started to cry. Matthew, who also seemed to have become attached to her, asked her in all seriousness: "Why don't you come with us?" He is now twenty but wouldn't have been surprised if she had said "yes" and had actually come. To him this would have been perfectly normal. He was delighted to be back home, stroked our cat very delicately, looked fondly at the goldfish in the aquarium and asked me if I had fed them regularly, and kept repeating about his time at the NIH: "It was good, though. It was great!"

Chapter Twelve

Matthew's Sense of Humor

Matthew liked riddles—the straightforward kind. Those that were more complex, which often must be worked out spontaneously, immediately, effortlessly, on the basis of implicit references within the vast system of signs—body language, expression, context, voice, tone, and inflection—on which social communication relies, posed problems that to him were insoluble, and of which he was in any case serenely unaware. From a very young age, he had enjoyed nursery rhymes, "Humpty Dumpty" for instance; when I would ask him who Humpty Dumpty was, he would always answer gladly "an egg" (he never tired of hearing that question and of repeating that answer). It was perfectly natural to him that *"All the king's horses/And all the king's men/Couldn't put Humpty Dumpty/Back together again."* He was amused by the idea that horses—even the horses of a king—were unable to put a broken egg together again. There were certain jokes he particularly liked, especially absurdist ones and those based on word play: these made him rock with happy laughter. He also was eager to tell such jokes and make others laugh. He liked reversal of word meanings in well-known phrases or other micro-verbal contexts—not longer than a sentence or two. Absurdity was something he naturally enjoyed, especially when it came in the form of simple, childish rhymes that he easily remembered. He was happy to listen to or recite nursery rhymes even in his early twenties. With him I rediscovered the inexpressible charm of these playful ditties, with improbable and apparently arbitrary imagery, but which—precisely because they are easily remembered—can in fact be applied to many life situations. (For example, the title of a book about Nixon, famous in its time, *All the President's Men*, was a transparent allusion to Humpty Dumpty's *"All the king's horses/And all the king's men,"* implying that after Watergate, Nixon's men—his staff, his counsel, his aides—could not possibly put him *"back together again,"* that he had been damaged beyond repair.)

There was a period, when Matthew was around sixteen or seventeen years old and had distanced himself from this type of infantile and poetic absurdism, when he would say in his most earnest tone, although perhaps with a touch of regret, "I'm no longer a baby. I'm a grownup. I'm not interested in that sort of thing." But later, he stopped minding. He must have been twenty or so when I bought—for him but also for myself, with my interest in the stylistic aspects of these gently absurdist short poems—*The Oxford Book of Nursery Rhymes,* a volume with critical notes and historical explanations, from which I sometimes read aloud to him. He listened with delight, and also with a more mature critical sense that did not, however, spoil his enjoyment of that particular type of childish humor. I fully shared in his delight. For him, this may have represented a chance to return to his childhood, to the level of his arrested emotional age, a return sanctioned by me, his almost omniscient father, the adult *par excellence* from his perspective. We spent long hours this way, with him proudly showing me that he still remembered and could recite the verses which I used to read aloud to him when he was little from *Mother Goose Rhymes,* a volume long lost or mislaid. I was amazed, knowing what a bad memory he had, by this awakening of recollections from a slumber of many years. One might argue that this was a case of mere mechanical recollection, radically different from that involuntary Proustian memory of "time regained"; but couldn't it also have been for Matthew an access path, a mode of reviving long-past

instants of luminous, ineffable bliss from his childhood? Involuntary recollection by means of rote memory? Difficult to say.

At work, Matthew often invented humorous riddles for his workmates
and, when he was in a good mood, did the same at home for us. Inspired,
for instance, by a program on the Nickelodeon channel for youngsters,
where someone asked the question "Why did the one-eyed monster close
down his school?" the answer being "Because he had only one pupil," he
created other similar literalist-playful riddles: "Why did the one-eyed
monster close his 'Barber's shop'?" The answer: "Because its sign had no
'i'." Or: "Why did the one-eyed monster close his 'Movie Cinema'?" Answer: "Because it had two 'i's." Of course, variations such as these, based
on homonyms, become quite obscure, even hermetic, because the absence
of the letter "i" in a trade sign has no apparent connection with the word
"eye" (as "pupil" does) or with the single eye of the fictional monster in
the initial riddle. Even more difficult to grasp was Matthew's connection
between the two "i"s in "Movie Cinema," which are not even pronounced
in the same way as the alphabet letter "i" and cannot, therefore, suggest the
phonetic homonymy "i" = *eye*. Some of Matthew's riddles were based on
such literalist or, shall I say, autistic strangeness, but he was always ready to
explain them and then people smiled or laughed, initially at his convoluted
explanations and subsequently at the ingenuity of his associations.

Other types of humor in Matthew's arsenal were based on shifts of
clichés (for instance, Egypt = the Sphinx). Thus, Georgianne told him one
day that she had received a phone call from Egypt. "Do you want to go to
Egypt?" Matthew asked her, adding: "Do you want to take the Sphinx's
place?" (Did he say this because he perceived Georgianne as a Sphinx-like,
mysterious person?)

It was also Georgianne who persuaded him to go to Dr. B., a dentist-
surgeon, to have his wisdom teeth removed, something he greatly feared.
She told Matthew—creating a wild scenario in order to motivate him—that
he could help her marry Dr. B., with whom she was in love. If he agreed
to go with her, the doctor, who loved her too but was extremely shy, might
use that opportunity to propose. She knew that Matthew would believe
her cockeyed story. Kind and generous as he was, Matthew was keen to

help. They both tried to find a workable stratagem for Matthew, who was ready to sacrifice his wisdom teeth for the cause, to convince the dentist that Georgianne was worth marrying. With this objective in mind, he started asking Georgianne a series of naïvely indiscreet questions such as: "How many showers do you have each week? How many times do you wash your face each day?" After she answered, somewhat bewildered, Matthew said decisively: "I'm going to tell Doctor B. that my friend Georgianne is a wonderful person, that she showers every day and washes her face twice daily." Which he actually did, to the doctor's amused confusion. Once he had delivered that statement, Matthew meekly allowed his wisdom teeth to be removed without protest or the slightest sign of fear. As he and Georgianne left, he mumbled to himself, without really expecting a reaction or response: "Georgianne is a wonderful person." This was humorous-autistic chivalry, Matthew-style.

There were many other similarly odd stories I have forgotten. But it was clear to me that Matthew had an innate sense of the absurd. He felt familiar with absurdity, integrating it without difficulty in the fabric of everyday life. Absurdity may have seemed to him more normal than normality, and free from banality or triviality—above all verbal triteness—which irritated him. This was why trivial dinner-time conversations—comments about food, such as: "This food is really nice, isn't it?" and the like—were met with hostile silence. I had learned my lesson: when he fell silent, I tried to say something unusual, something likely to attract his attention, something unexpected, perhaps a joke—even when I didn't feel like joking and when, amidst all my worries, I would have found small talk welcome and relaxing. In such circumstances my jokes were most of the time well received, dragging Matthew out of his stubborn silence and encouraging him to joke in his turn. Unfortunately, however, on many such evenings this tactic had no effect: no, his silence was not really hostile, he simply felt unwell, perhaps he had a migraine (a long-standing problem), or was in one of those states preceding a seizure. On such occasions, we dined in silence. I knew something was not right but did not want to pester him with questions, because questions only made things worse, and in any case he never wanted to talk about how he felt. He wanted to talk only when he felt fine.

Matthew's type of absurdist humor reminded me of Eugène Ionesco's first play, *The Bald Soprano*. Some time ago I read a review in the *New York Times* of a production of this play by an avant-garde director whose name now escapes me. I thought his concept was original and plausible, given the possibilities of ambiguity of the absurd. The cliché-ridden dialogues between Mr. Smith and Mrs. Smith and especially those between the Martins—who discover to their amazement that they inhabit the same house, are married, and have children—were no longer treated as a satire of petty bourgeois mediocrity (as they were in most productions), but as tragically humorous exchanges between autistics or amnesiacs or schizophrenics, offering an unexpected new perspective on Ionesco's own definition of the play as a "tragedy of language." A very comic tragedy, indeed, which makes you laugh throughout, but which nevertheless remains a tragedy of a certain alienated human condition, if not of the human condition in general. Having read the review, I would have liked to see this off-off-Broadway production but, obviously, it was bound to have a very short run and it was no longer on when I went to New York later on.

Chapter Thirteen

At 20: The Ages of Matthew, from *Diary about Matthew* (1997)

In the summer of 1997, a few days before Matthew's twentieth birthday and a couple of months before the trip to NIH, I wrote in *Diary about Matthew:*

❋ What most worries me is the constant, almost inexorable increase in frequency of Matthew's seizures. They have become noticeably shorter—from two, three, even four minutes a few years ago to thirty to forty seconds now—but they occur not only more often but at random intervals. [In the course of 1997 he had forty-six seizures that we could observe and who knows how many, possibly less intense, that passed unnoticed. In 1998, there were fifty-nine.] They are more frequent, more unpredictable, more frightening.

His speech difficulties have also become more serious. Whenever he wants to say something, he searches painfully and helplessly for words. It almost physically pains me to hear his prolonged struggle to articulate words, a struggle that can last up to one long minute. In the end he manages to utter only a few hesitant words, and these often have no grammatical or logical connection and remain, therefore, incomprehensible. The meaning of whatever it is that he wants to communicate is clear in his mind (his face shows that he is bewildered by our incomprehension), but his message does not come across, it remains unintelligible. It is probably something very simple and, in order to help him, we try to do a bit of guesswork, but our responses to his involuntary riddles are mostly off the mark and, in frustration, he gives up, with his usual expression of irritated and astonished frustration: "Never mind! Never mind!" On the rare occasions when we do guess what he wants to say, he seems to take it as perfectly natural. He seems to believe that the people he is talking to, his mother and father, and others too, are fully aware of his intentions and of whatever he is painfully trying to say, but inexplicably pretend not to understand. If he really suffers from what clinical psychologists call mind-blindness—the failure to read plausibly the minds of others—the opposite could also be true in Matthew's case. It could well be that he believes his mind is transparent, that his thoughts can be read by others, that in fact they can be seen directly, which would render language, so difficult for him to handle, completely redundant. He enjoys being talked to, being told real or imaginary stories, which he listens to in silence, especially if they are told in everyday, colloquial language. Naïvely, he seems to imagine that we actually know what he means when he speaks. His exasperated "Never mind" sounds like a reproach, and causes us much pain. We continue to go through a complex process of inference and speculation, because in fact we do not have an external clue, a common referential framework or any other lead. If he finds it difficult, or even impossible, to read us, we find it equally difficult to read him. What is clear is that he needs and loves us—the common view that autistic people have no feelings is false—and that we love him, possibly not in the same way, but as much. We know that we must hide our love for him to accept it and feel reassured by it.

Last year he insisted on going to university and, with the aid of private tutors and constant help from us, he managed to take two courses (one per semester) and pass his final exams, with a B in English composition and a C+ in pre-calculus. (Was this because the talent for math he had shown in primary school and then in middle and high school was limited, or because he had regressed?) These courses, although of little value to him academically, were a good way for him to spend his time, to somehow fill its emptiness. I mean by this mainly social time, time he spent with his private tutors, themselves students, good, understanding, patient youngsters who came to our house several times a week and whom Matthew always awaited with eagerness. He likes them and they seem to like him, too. He enjoys being with people who help him and explain things to him calmly and gently: in such situations, he always does his best, focuses and, more importantly, understands. But although he understands quite clearly, it is only for a short time, after which he forgets, so that the results of this work—a labor of love while it lasts—are nil. Work is not something he does with a long-term view—the future exists for him only as a nonfuture, something he avoids thinking of, something even dangerous to think about. Work for him has meaning only as a pleasant way to pass time, which would otherwise be hollow, restless, pointless; work for him is an end in itself, ephemeral, leaving no trace. Matthew lives almost exclusively in the present: almost without exception he seems to push his past experiences if not into total oblivion, at least into some gray area, a space in which only a very powerful searchlight—a special art of remembrance that we, his parents, have come to practice quite often—can pick out the occasional random memory: "Ah, yes, I remember now!"

Over the last two years he has been working—three afternoons per week—at a university center that sends questionnaires to high school students in Indiana, especially to those from poorer families, offering them college grants on the condition that they graduate on time. Matthew is responsible for arranging files alphabetically, a difficult and tedious job given that hundreds of replies arrive regularly in the mail, but a job Matthew performs with minute precision, much valued by his colleagues, mainly students paid hourly like himself. They are aware of his handicap and treat him well, like a "normal" person, joke with him and laugh sincerely at his strange little jokes, showing him much affection. He is thriving in this atmosphere, he feels happy. From what his colleagues say, he experiences fewer speech difficulties at work. His unexpected verbal associations, absurdly illogical but always containing a hidden logic, produce general merriment, in which he too takes part. Some of his jokes are similar to the one he used with Dr. Leventhal in Chicago, who saw him in 1989, one I've never been able to erase from memory. "When's your birthday?" the doctor asked him, and he said: "7 + 5 + 20 – 6 – 2 August," which was exactly 24 August, but expressed in a childishly convoluted way.

Matthew seems to be different ages simultaneously, to have attained several levels of development, all of them lagging behind what is normally expected of a young man of twenty. His emotional age is that of a four- or five-year-old, or even someone younger—and for me this is the core of his being, the source of his innocence as well as of his mysterious fragility. This could explain why he is most comfortable in the company of young children, with whom he plays readily, enjoying their presence, their endearingly clumsy gestures, their laughter and bewilderment, to which he adds his own. When someone visits with a small child, Matthew rushes to the room where he keeps his huge collection of stuffed animals, bringing them out one by one and placing them in front of the child. Sometimes he will demonstrate how to play with a small toy monkey and then offer it and sit still, gazing at the child in silent and fascinated contemplation. If it is a toddler asleep in its stroller, he remains motionless, staring, oblivious of time. In such situations, he does not realize how strange an image he projects: a young, tall, well-built male of twenty, kneeling in front of a baby carriage watching its occupant with utter seriousness or, if the child is awake, trying to catch its attention with a toy.

Matthew's social age is that of a pre-teen, passionate about sports. He can watch sports events on TV endlessly and read about them with undivided attention in the morning, in the local paper or in *USA Today*. He has a complete grasp of sports vocabulary and can discuss any of the most popular sports such as baseball, football, basketball, tennis knowledgeably with fans. His expertise extends to sports with a more limited local audience, such as ice hockey or soccer. Matthew's age as a reader is also pre-teen: in a more general sense, whenever he reads for pleasure—which he does rarely—he reads books for youngsters or the occasional biography of a famous athlete. His sexual life is at the same pre-teen level: his interests in this respect are marginal, barely observable, if not altogether absent.

(Freud, too, noted the period of indifference between infant sexuality, so intense up to about five years of age, and the reawakening of the libido in adolescence.) Matthew has the odd wet dream, but is otherwise completely removed from matters of a sexual nature. He is naturally chaste, even in his language—he never uses dirty words and reacts reproachfully when others use them in his presence. How intense Matthew's sexuality as a child might have been I do not know, but I tend to think that the medication he has been taking for more than six years now must have weakened his sexual impulses. As for his mental age, it is close to a sixteen- or seventeen-year-old's when he focuses and really wants to understand something, but, as I have said, he quickly forgets everything. Perhaps he doesn't see the point of keeping such knowledge alive in his memory. Or, perhaps, here too, it is the effect of medication.

Apart from his mentor from Harmony School, Phil Wheeler, his only other friend is Julian. He appears to be very different from Matthew and could actually be taken for any average eighteen-year-old. In total contrast to Matthew, Julian is a good speaker—fluent, rapid, using vivid colloquial language full of idiomatic expressions. I would even say that Julian is a persuasive speaker: not so long ago, he got a job as a retail salesman with Cutco, a firm that sells quality, expensive knives of various types. When he came to the house with a kit of knives with shiny blades, I asked for a demonstration of his sales pitch, and was so impressed with his performance that I immediately bought two kitchen knives that cost ten times more than I would have paid in an ordinary store, and for which I had no need whatsoever.

I sometimes wonder: how can a young man as articulate as Julian, articulate but possibly not highly intelligent, spend such long hours with Matthew? Why does he drive 220 miles to Bloomington from Chicago, where he moved with family a couple of years ago, in order to spend a weekend with Matthew? (Matthew does not drive and cannot obtain a driver's license because of his epilepsy, but I doubt he would be able to drive even if he did not suffer from that condition.) It is a mystery to me. It is true that Julian also suffers from autism or Asperger's syndrome, but he is developmentally more advanced than Matthew, and socially much more sophisticated. I tell myself that, in spite of his apparent social abilities, Julian is probably the same age as Matthew emotionally. That must be why they get along so well. There is no other way to explain the affection that binds them, or the fact that Julian has no other close friends—real friends, as opposed to casual acquaintances—among his peers. Interestingly, he too seems to have no interest whatsoever in girls, romance, or erotic experiences. The secret child in Julian is well-hidden—much better hidden than in Matthew—but no less real. Matthew's comes out whenever he gets a chance, in all his naïve earnestness (the younger Matthew is very timid and rarely smiles, unlike his older self).

Last summer we took Matthew to Paris to meet his family there, my sister Ina and her husband Petre, as well as their daughter, Claudia, married to the lawyer Jean-Pierre Ghestin and mother to little Edouard, my sixteen-month-old nephew and godson, who is thus a second cousin to Matthew. Once, we all went for a walk in the small park not far from the apartment, on Boulevard Raspail, where the Ghestins live. There were other children in the park, and Matthew was purely and simply carried away. He started playing in the sand with Edouard's little spade and bucket, with the earnest expression of someone in an algebra class. Uca and I felt rather embarrassed. Another time, when the three of us—Uca, Matthew, and I— went down to the Bois de Boulogne, we entered the Jardin d'acclimatation, a children's amusement park with miniature trains, ponies, a funhouse with distorting mirrors, and other attractions. It was a Sunday morning and the visitors were mostly parents or nannies with children under the age of twelve. Matthew was in heaven. "This park is for young children," I told him, trying to convince him that we should move on to the Bagatelle, famous for its flowers and especially for its roses, then in full season. Impossible. Matthew was in his element and didn't want to leave.

Phil Wheeler said this about Matthew's friend Julian, when he visited a few days ago: "Julian hasn't got the faintest idea about what's going on in the world; he is just as disoriented as I was before they diagnosed me with autism; he doesn't understand that he does not understand and has no idea if he is doing the right thing or not. He is completely lost." By which

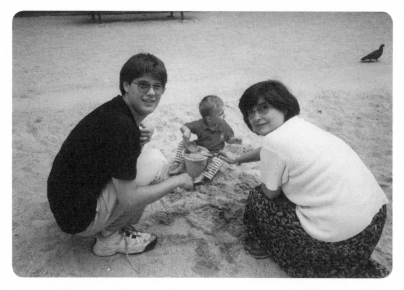

Playing in the Jardin d'acclimatation, Paris, 1997 (age 20)

he might have meant: Matthew, for one, understands that Julian does not understand. This is perhaps the reason for their friendship. This may also be Matthew's "wisdom."

What worries me, as I have already said, is less the autism (with which we are becoming reconciled) than his uncontrollable epileptic seizures, and the medication which is supposed to reduce their frequency, but which cannot fail to have side effects. Only two days ago he had two seizures, one in the early morning as he was still asleep (it was not too intense and lasted for only about thirty seconds) and the other one in the evening, around five minutes to ten, shortly after he had gone to bed. He was very tired after the day's trip to Indianapolis, where he went with his co-workers Mary Anne, Amy, Courtney, and Heather to help file correspondence at the Center's IUPUI (Indiana University–Purdue University in Indianapolis) branch. The next day I asked him if he'd felt tired in the van on the way home, after such a full day. I wanted to take down his exact words. "I did feel tired on the way back," he told me, slightly suspicious. "Are you writing this down, or what? No, I don't think I fell asleep." (He is aware that the seizures occur in his sleep.) "I just lay like this"—and he stretched on the sofa in the TV room with half-closed eyes. "Then I opened my eyes and we talked. Are you writing all this down to show to Dr. Wisen? Don't show him. Perhaps it's true, perhaps not, I don't know." Could he have had a seizure (probably a minor one) on the minibus, a seizure that nobody had noticed and of which he himself was only half-aware, and wanted to keep it a secret? Is he afraid that the doctor, if informed, might reach the wrong conclusion? Dr. Wisen is a supremely authoritative figure for him, and he would not want him to be misled. Perhaps it is true, perhaps not. For Matthew truth must be true in the strictest sense of the term. He hates deception of any kind. He would not want things he is not sure about to pass for truth.

Chapter Fourteen

When Matthew Was 25 . . .

I could always recognize him at a distance, unmistakably, even in a crowd of people milling about: he was tall, broad-shouldered, strong and yet vulnerable, with long hands and very long fingers (a condition known as acromegaly in medicine), long legs, a strange, cautious walk, unhurried, swaying slightly from side to side. Unaware that I was observing him as I drew nearer, he usually wore an earnest, thoughtful expression on his unshaven face, with an ever-present, almost imperceptible incipient smile to himself, ready to bloom if he met someone he knew. Then, his beautiful hazel eyes lighted up with a short-lived flicker of awakened attention before softening back into their normal contemplative gaze of gentle melancholy. If we bumped into each other accidentally, in the street or in some shop at the College Mall, where he would spend a lot of time (in the Borders book-store, for instance, where he could linger for an hour or more after work, browsing through videotapes and more recently DVDs) he was genuinely surprised and pleased for a few moments, after which he became worried that I might ask him to come home, when all he wanted was to be left on his own, free to return home when he chose, taking his time strolling along in his swaying walk, lost in his own thoughts, smiling to himself.

He was, at twenty-five, a particularly good-looking young man, with gracefully arched eyebrows beneath his glasses, which he had been wearing for many years due to astigmatism. He had rich, light-chestnut hair and eyes with a golden glitter in the sunshine. He looked disheveled without actually being so, the soft skin of his face with a stubble which he allowed to grow for days or even a week or two because, with his awkward movements and his very sensitive skin, shaving was a minor torture which he kept postponing. He dressed casual-smart like most youngsters these days, but with an almost obsessive concern for cleanliness: he would never wear a shirt, or more commonly, a T-shirt, longer than a day; even his jeans, or trousers—the faded sort, of which he had dozens—had to be washed frequently, every two days, not because they were dirty, but because they had to have that fresh feel, that smell of freshly laundered cloth so crucial for his extraordinary olfactory sensitivity. (He was so totally, almost violently intolerant of the faintest whiff of cigarette smoke that I gave up smoking altogether, while Uca had her few daily cigarettes, which she was reluctant to give up, outdoors, in the backyard, even in the most stifling summer heat or the harshest of winter chills.)

Matthew had changed in many ways, but had remained the same in many others. He had become a more tolerant grownup, respecting our time and our obligations. He never woke us up in the morning, although he occasionally got up with the birds; he let us work when we told him we needed to. He was keen on having serious talks with Uca and, more recently, even with me. He continued to be highly moral and responsible, as he had been from early on, but with less of his former rigidity; he had also become more sociable, had even learned to lie on occasion, albeit half-heartedly and with a shy tentativeness that often betrayed him. He practiced his absurdist humor, his bizarre jokes, as a way of being social, and was happy when he could make others laugh—building on and valorizing some of his mental inabilities, such as his tendency to literalism, as comic sources.

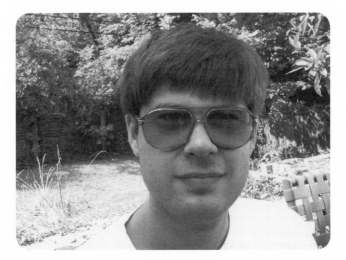

Birthday portrait, 2002

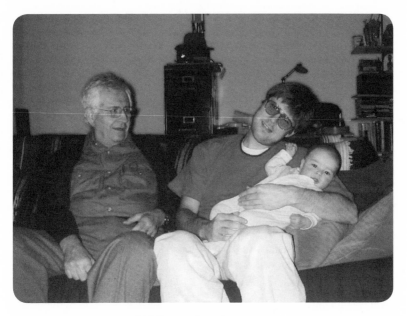

Holding nephew Rory, 2002

I find it interesting, and worth noting here, that his latest favorite film was *Bicentennial Man,* based on a sci-fi story by Isaac Asimov. He had seen it at the theater and subsequently bought the DVD, and he watched it repeatedly. The story is set in a distant future, yet in a world very similar to today's America in terms of social ambience, family life, and human reactions. It features a couple with two daughters in a typical American home and a domestic labor-saving robot, bought in a store, which gradually becomes human. An early scene shows the robot asking the man of the house, who is sympathetic toward him, to tell a joke. The man tells him a few funny anecdotes, which the robot commits to memory. In a later scene, in the garden, the robot surprises the mother and the two daughters by reciting these anecdotes in an automatic monotone, without pausing for the punch line: the three women listen to him attentively in increasing bewilderment, and burst out laughing uncontrollably at the end. The robot is elated: this newly acquired ability to make others laugh is a great step toward its humanization. Finally the robot becomes human to such an extent that he gives up his immortality in exchange for being recognized as a full-fledged man. Exactly at that moment he dies, because he is suddenly very old, two hundred years old (hence the title). In the meantime, Matthew had stopped believing that all movies are good. He liked some, disliked others, while still others remained in the gray area, which Stine Levy said was inaccessible to autistic people. In the process of becoming an adult, Matthew had acquired the ability to formulate value judgments, to be sensitive to nuances, even when he found it difficult to describe them in other than general terms. The scene in which Andrew-the-robot becomes fully human and dies as a consequence fascinated him.

He had retained the serenity and charm that were already on full display as early as his Harmony School days. On his way home, or making a slight detour, he still used to drop by his old school, where he seemed to have left his heart. He was as welcome there as he had been in the early days, when we had moved him there from the public school. He chatted with his former teachers, met the new ones, and was visibly delighted to watch the children as they stormed past him in the corridors, or in the garden during breaks. I remember that Bart, his shop teacher, and Matthew once dismantled an old bicycle and reassembled it with the missing pieces purchased from a second-hand bicycle store, so that in the end it looked like new; the students all gathered at the windows of the school's two-story building to applaud and cheer him as he took the first triumphal tour. Julie, one of the teachers, later purchased the bike for a minimal sum, which was donated to the school.

A few words about the school. The old building, located in our neighborhood, had been a public elementary school, which was abandoned when the school moved into the newer Rogers and Binford buildings. The community put the old school building up for sale for the symbolic sum of one dollar on the condition that it be used for educational purposes. Harmony had functioned for a few years in another neighborhood as a private alternative school. Named after an early-nineteenth-century utopian community in Indiana, it was organized by a group of young left-wing teachers, trained in the 1960s—the years of student revolt and anti-war protests—for the benefit of children who, for various reasons, could not or did not want to attend public schools.

For Matthew this school was a blessing. Fees were fixed according to parents' incomes, and poorer children were accepted free. The environment was entirely non-competitive, relaxed, permissive, but not at all irresponsible. The school encouraged creativity: for example, end-of-year festivities featured many improvised events organized by the children themselves, who were also in charge of bringing out the school yearbook. Teachers knew every student well, and children with difficulties were given special attention, with curricular activities tailored to their needs. Based on egalitarian principles, the school encouraged students to learn according to their own abilities and interests, but, curiously enough, their scores at standardized tests were high and Harmony managed to maintain its accreditation. In its own way it was an experimental school where, in my view, one did not learn much. For the advanced grade levels, we moved Matthew to High School South, a public high school with hundreds if not thousands of students, which we thought might prepare him better for the future.

But, no matter how implausible it may sound, Matthew did in fact

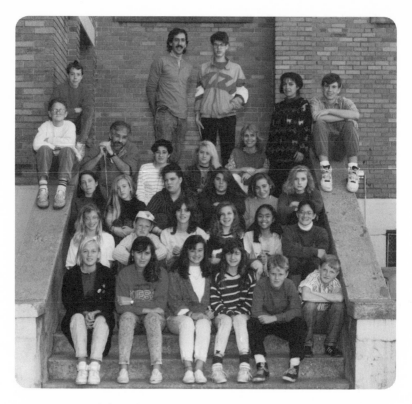

*In eighth grade at Harmony, 1990 (back row, standing,
with teacher Daniel Baron) (age 13)*

learn a good deal at Harmony. In the first place, he learned how to freely
exercise his charm over others—his frail but highly efficient weapon. He
learned to be kind, to repress his violent impulses, to block out whatever
was bothering or disconcerting him and wait patiently for the situation to
improve. The teachers devised three modes of "walking-as-punishment" to
help him calm down when he felt angry: up and down the corridor, around
the school building or, if he had been very disruptive, around the block.
Also at Harmony, owing to the special care of his teachers, he got to meet
Phil Wheeler, recruited by the school as a voluntary tutor for one of its
students with autism. This was to be a crucial encounter in Matthew's life.

Even from an academic viewpoint, he learned many things—which, it is true, he promptly forgot, as he forgot most of what he learned, even things that he grasped firmly when he first learned them (like complex math and pre-calculus). Possibly because he could only live and think in the present, uncomfortable with the idea of time, possibly because he did not want or could not—owing to his otherworldly or angelic nature?—fall into time, he lacked the ability to connect what he understood so clearly one day to what was about to happen the next. He lacked what I would call the cumulative faculty of the human mind. He did not forget because he had a poor memory—tests had shown that his memory was good—but because he had no sense of time or because he rejected time. A fundamental human deficiency, but possibly also, for someone like him, an inexpressible gift. His years at Harmony were probably his most carefree and happy, which is why he was so glad to go back again, after long years. He enjoyed the relaxed, informal, friendly atmosphere, in which students would address their teachers in a familiar way, by their first names; and he liked to roam through the old building, less functional than modern schools but so full of character that Matthew, enchanted by it, included it in his little grateful speech at the end of his last year there.

As I have already suggested, on a deeper level Matthew had remained unchanged. He could easily switch to the sensibility of a third- or fourth-grader. His emotional age (a non-scientific concept) had remained at his third, fourth, or fifth year. That is something only other autistic people could fully sense or intuit. Of course, in the meantime he had learned he had autism, and he was happy to attend the monthly dinners of the group of young autistic people in Bloomington, named ABLES and organized by three admirable women: Suzi Rimstidt, a mother, Susan Grey, a social worker, and Nancy Dalrymple, a researcher. We also took him to various conferences on autism, where he was interested almost exclusively in the presentations by people like him—some famous in the small world of autism, such as Donna Williams or Temple Grandin—or in meeting fellow autistics, with whom he established instant friendships that he maintained long afterward, largely by phone but also by e-mail. On one such occasion he made the acquaintance of Ann Hendrickson, a thirty-four-year-old woman from Indianapolis who worked in one of the administrative departments of the state of Indiana, and with whom he talked regularly on the phone, at least once a week, for hours. He also met Scott Bales from Atlanta, a surveyor at the Cartographic Institute of the state of Georgia, of whom he became very fond and with whom he remained in constant touch by phone or e-mail, as he did with Julian. With these people he communicated in a language beyond ordinary language: a mysterious, wordless, exhilarating means of connectedness, mind to mind and soul to soul.

Chapter Fifteeen

Julian's Visit

Julian came from New Jersey to visit us after Matthew's death. He couldn't make it to the service, but he came a few days later and stayed with us for four days. He slept in the TV room, the room in which Matthew had passed away. As a friend, it may have given him a kind of melancholy pleasure, reinforcing a sense of intimacy, not altogether lost—just as I loved wearing Matthew's sleeveless gray vest, in which I sensed a trace of his warm body, a hint of his presence, which somehow rendered him tangible. People are generally reluctant to sleep in the bed of someone who has recently died, or wear their clothes. But, as well as the gray vest, I seek out Matthew's clothes and wear those that fit me. I wear them with love (this is the precise word), with a sad serenity, as if by doing so I come closer to his shade, to his affectionate memory, so vivid yet so distant, beyond the reach of words. The other day, as it was quite cold, I put on the leather jacket we bought him at the onset of winter, though we feared he might refuse to wear it because he generally did not like gifts or new things. He would scold us for wasting money on him, he who needed nothing, who could wear the same clothes for years without minding.

But he liked that leather jacket and accepted it, not because it looked good, but because it was soft and smooth to the touch, because his fingers felt a cool thrill when he caressed it—the same way he used to lightly stroke Mikadoo, our cat who died three years ago, holding her in his lap for hours, delicately touching her fur and listening to her purr. Strangely enough, he didn't miss her when she died, didn't ask about her. But sometimes when he touched a soft surface he was reminded of her, and he was sad when he called and she did not come, even though he knew she had died. He liked that jacket so much that he was reluctant to wear it, afraid it might get stolen at the public library where he worked. He used to leave his winter things in a combination-locker, but he quite illogically lost confidence in the locker after the small pouch in which he kept his wallet, ID, and house key was stolen—not, however, from the locker, but from the library's public toilet where he had left it for just a few minutes. From that moment on, he was careful to keep his belongings with him: his coat, hat, and, on snowy winter days, his boots—on those days he took his sneakers with him to wear at the library. Even so, he feared losing that jacket. Finally I convinced him to hang it in the librarians' cloakroom, and of course nobody stole it from there. Eventually I "stole" it from him myself, wearing it and stroking it in his memory, sensing the shape of his body, which it had fit so elegantly—although I was too heavy for it and left it unbuttoned to disguise the fact. I didn't want to look ridiculous in the street—whereas he wouldn't have cared less. I have been wearing that almost new leather jacket for a few days now and will be wearing it again and again on cold days, thinking of him.

Julian, soberly dressed now—in a short rainproof jacket, far from new, and the eternal T-shirt and basketball shoes commonly worn by youngsters, with blondish, undyed hair (the Mohawk hairdo and the bicycle chain around his neck now live on only in my memory)—embraced us timidly, barely uttering the conventional condolences in a low, pained, near-whisper: he had lost his great friend. What was he doing these days? He worked part-time in a halfway house for schizophrenics and other mentally ill people in New Jersey. He was hoping to get a full-time job there in the future. It was—he admitted—not a very cheerful job, but it was OK. Did he have a relationship, a girlfriend? No, but he did take this girl out now and then, though he wasn't getting on with her all that well. Why? Because whenever someone starts getting too close to him, he has a tendency to withdraw.

Did he have any friends? Not really. Obviously, he cared for some of his former schoolmates from Harmony, among them Austin and Andy, who still live in Bloomington and whom he was going to see. But Matthew had been his great friend. How had the two of them been getting along—on the phone—lately? Great! But not because of what they said; *it was an understanding,* he explained without really explaining, though his meaning was clear for me: it was an understanding beyond words. It was, I thought, enough for them to hear each other's voice, to chat about sports and sport results, about everything and nothing; what mattered was the heard voice, the expected, recollected, renewed vocal contact, the rest did not really matter. What he told me brought me once more up against the mystery of communication between people with autism, and especially with Asperger's syndrome. I believe that what is important here is a profoundly human element: knowing for sure that someone expects nothing from you apart from the simple fact of your *being* there, existing; knowing that they are not interested in the information you can give them, or in the favors you can do them, or in creating a sympathy that you might want reciprocated in the way you value them; knowing that you value them not for the smart or original things they can tell you, but simply because they are like you. For two people to have this certitude is what I would call a pure, disinterested friendship, at the level of pure being: it does not matter what you *have* to offer me, but who you *are*.

This is why Julian was so affected by Matthew's death: he was the Friend, as Julian was, for Matthew, the Friend, although not the only one. As for Julian, who functions almost like ordinary people verbally and socially, who has no contacts with other autistics and does not attend conferences on this topic, his chances of meeting someone like Matthew again are minimal, if not altogether nonexistent. (There are apparently no people with autism at the halfway house where he works now.) He and Matthew met as children and established a relationship that lasted for years, in spite of life's ups and downs. The continuity of their relationship was what mattered for both of them.

Interestingly, both Julian and Matthew became vegetarians at some stage, about ten years ago. But while Julian became a vegan, Matthew kept milk, eggs, cheese, and fish in his diet; he would not have touched meat for anything in the world, although as a child he had relished hamburgers, which Uca and I detested. Both of them described their adoption of vegetarianism as a life philosophy (compassion for the animals brutally killed in slaughterhouses), but I think that in Matthew's case, at least, the repulsion he felt for meat came also from deeper physiological causes. It was a bodily intolerance, which in my view was due to the fact that some of the substances in meat actually made him ill. His own body had become the invisible inner doctor who ordered him to avoid meat of any kind, with the exception of fish. Could this self-imposed prohibition have had any link with his autism or epilepsy? The fact is he became a vegetarian when he started having epileptic seizures. When I asked Dr. Patterson, the neurologist at Mayo, if there could be a link between his seizures and his abstinence from meat (in the sense of a defense reaction of the organism, a sign that could be worth considering for the benefit of a better diagnosis and better targeted dietary measures in the future), he told me confidently that no, there was no link. Personally, I was not convinced; I continue to believe that this obscure link has not yet been discovered and systematically studied.

In spite of all the precautions recommended by Matthew's inner doctor, his seizures became steadily more serious. They—and the medication prescribed to combat them—had serious side effects, observable over time. His capacity for verbal expression had deteriorated, compared to his abilities at the age of seven or eight, when he had been diagnosed with autism. Comparatively, at that age he spoke well, with a certain vivacity even, as we noticed in a videotape from that period that we watched again, first with Julian and then with Phil Wheeler and his family, after Matthew's death. Likewise his short-term memory deteriorated, as we had noticed. The miracle—if one may speak of miracles in such circumstances—was that there had been no change in his character, except positive change.

His character was beautiful from the start, in spite of the misfortunes that struck him, and became increasingly beautiful, painfully beautiful for us: he was tolerant but discerning at the same time, endowed with a kindness that radiated from the midst of his silent suffering, a kindness that could increasingly be taken for happiness. In this fundamental sense Matthew was, I think, happy: the absurd prediction that I wrote down in my old diary a few days after he was born came true. It did not come true as we would have wished, but it came abundantly true, for us and for him, in that gentle light of his kindness, which shone and still shines on us.

Chapter Sixteen

Questions without an Answer

Perhaps the only enlightening truism of the many that are uttered about death is this: when you die, you become as you were before you were born. Matthew, of course, especially as a teenager, used to ask me about death, and when I repeated this phrase to him he was perplexed. "What do you mean, as I was before I was born?" "Well, the way you were, let's say, in 1973, when we left Romania and came to America." "At that stage," he said, jokingly, "I was minus four years old, wasn't I? But what was I like then?" "I don't know, Matthew, I really don't know. If I knew, I would tell you." "But did I exist then?" "Who knows?" "What about God, doesn't he know?" "Maybe he does, but we can't ask him, because he doesn't answer questions." "He doesn't answer questions? Why don't you answer then? What is death?" I kept repeating the same old cliché: "It's how you were before you were born. Try to imagine that." This was usually the end of our conversations about death. Matthew would fall into silent thought; but sometimes he would ask—and his question was in fact a form of affirmation, a rhetorical question, a kind of certitude: "What about heaven?" (Some Christian heretics, followers of Origen, believed that souls existed before birth, before gaining an earthly corporeality, and continued to exist, most certainly, after death, until the end of time, when all will be absorbed into divine eternity, when everybody, including the Devil, will finally be forgiven.)

Later, when he may have begun to have obscure premonitions of his own death, during such conversations—which normally took place in the evening, after dinner, when Matthew felt like talking and asking questions (possibly miming curiosity to encourage conversation, as he was otherwise rarely curious about things)—this topic was systematically avoided; the topics of our post-dinner conversations were wide-ranging, but death was not among them. He could no longer bear even to hear the word *death,* and therefore he was no longer keen to go to church, although he was a believer—because, he told us, they talked too much about death there. I don't think he feared his own death, but he feared the future (which, as he well knew, ends in death), especially his future, in our absence. We sometimes talked to him about the possibility of his being left, after our passing away, on his own; we assured him that he wouldn't lack anything, that we had made sure he would inherit the house on Wylie Street, which he loved so much, and that he would have everything he needed. We suggested that Phil and his sons might look after him, and possibly also Irena, if he were willing to move to Los Angeles (which he was not at all keen to do). We almost managed to convince him, in order to put his mind to rest, that being young he had a long, good life in store and would certainly outlive us. But he refused to think of this; he refused to think of the future. He seemed to have reached the conclusion that death is better not talked about. Yet in all this time, unbeknown to us, he was approaching his own death, with increasing calm and serenity. He may have sensed something recently, and was advancing toward it in the contemplative frame of mind of someone who thinks that this subject should remain shrouded in silence.

But what did death mean to him, after all? Did he wish for it, unconsciously but deeply, in the way that I had wished for it consciously and superficially, so many times? In a way, to return to the commonplace with which I opened this fragment, death is like birth in that we know nothing about either, we remember nothing, we can anticipate nothing. Is there

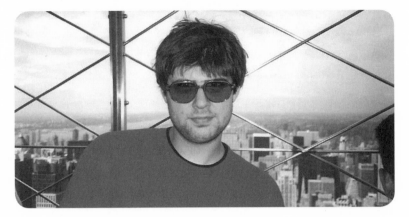

On the deck of the Empire State Building, New York City, 2002

merely an empty eternity before birth, and an empty eternity after death, between which life is a meaningless moment, or with at most a fleeting, purely imaginary significance, imparted to it by each one of us according to our powers, but ultimately signifying nothing (see *Ecclesiastes*)? Is life a miracle, as short-lived as any other, of no ultimate consequence? Jesus resurrected Lazarus, but did Lazarus not die in the end, like all of us? And how did Lazarus finally die? Why does the miracle of life itself, as the wise Solomon tells us in the bleakest and yet, to me, the most enlightening of all the books in the Bible, have no meaning? Are miracles by nature devoid of meaning? *Why, where to, what for?*

These are elementary queries in grammar. But what exists beyond these words? Beyond them lies only the kingdom of Chance, or of God. "A throw of the dice will never abolish chance . . . ," wrote Mallarmé. But there could be Something Else. *Perhaps*—a microscopic, but infinite, possibility. Matthew did believe in God, and in Jesus: unshaken in his faith, without fervor and without doubts, he had the simple, calm certainty that he was going to heaven.

BLOOMINGTON, MARCH–APRIL 2003

Postscript (2004)

Almost a year has passed since Matthew's death, and I have continued reading and thinking about autism and Asperger's syndrome as if he were alive.
I want to understand him, to understand his condition. Somehow he is still
around. The enigma he embodied haunts me and will do so for the rest of
my life. Curiously, epilepsy—which actually killed him—is not part of the
enigma. I wonder why? Perhaps because epilepsy, tragic and mysterious
as it may be, seems less perplexing than the autistic mind. And Matthew
survives in my memory not because of his heartbreaking and eventually
fatal seizure disorder, but because he was autistic, because he belonged to
that strange world, alien and yet, for all its apparent "otherness," tacitly—at
times desperately—demanding to be understood on its own terms, seeking empathy, not the normal kind (which it tends to reject), but cooler and
simpler, without gestures of compassion, less explicit or verbal, amenable
to silence, to the absence of context, to a sort of asocial or quasi-angelical
thinking (supposing that angels are mathematicians, preoccupied mostly
with resolving pure equations that have nothing to do with our real, com-

petitive, humanly ambitious world). Year after year I tried to understand Matthew, but only toward the end did I feel—rightly? wrongly?—that I was closer to him. This still did not mean that we could communicate—or, to use a better word, commune—in the more subtle ways he related to other autistic people. Those ways remained inaccessible to me.

Recently, reading Donna Williams's 1996 *Autism: An Inside-Out Approach,* I recalled the following episode, which illustrates indirectly and by contrast what I am trying to say. Some years ago, my wife and I attended a national conference organized by ASA (the Autism Society of America) in Indianapolis. We decided to take Matthew along because, aside from the usual professional lectures and panels, a few sessions were scheduled in which high-functioning autistics would share their life experience, and we thought that he would profit from listening to them. One of the featured speakers was Donna Williams, by then famous as author of the best-selling *Nobody Nowhere: The Extraordinary Autobiography of an Autistic* (1992). At her talk, I recall, Matthew was seated in the first row, in a full but completely silent room (the audience had been asked not to applaud, since the noise of clapping hands upset the frail-looking speaker). The silence was all the more necessary because Donna spoke in a trembling, feeble, barely audible voice, in a sort of *pianissimo* musical lisp. All ears, totally attentive, Matthew was staring at her with a happy look on his face. And Donna, noticing him, realized he was "like her." At the end of the talk she wanted to know the name of the tall, broad-shouldered young man with chestnut hair, in a T-shirt, wearing big glasses, sitting in the first row. The woman Donna spoke to (in a whisper) came straight up to Matthew and asked his name. She returned to Donna, then came back to him and said: "Donna says hi to Matthew!" Although he showed no sign of surprise, Matthew was obviously pleased and proud. I wonder whether he understood Donna's talk (being much less verbal than she was)—but did it actually matter? They recognized they shared the same world, and this recognition—achieved how?—erased all differences but of names. Matthew knew Donna's name, of course, but she needed to know his for that brief message of sheer recognition: "Donna says hi to Matthew." A message requiring no response (Matthew smiled to himself but said nothing), gratuitous but not devoid of a special kind of empathy, discreet and respectful of the other's solitary freedom, asking none of the reactions that social empathy normally entails. Instinctively, for an instant, Matthew and Donna had recognized each other—without any consequence. But are recognitions less true if they lack consequence?

I cannot help being intrigued by the ways in which autistics, unlike ordinary people, spontaneously and unfailingly recognize each other. Donna Williams writes: "This is a bit like an animal sensing whether another creature is of the same or related species or not. Some animals do this by smell or sound. Some animals certainly seem able to observe the foreignness and incomprehensibility of the behavior of creatures that are not like themselves [...]. When I am around non-autistic people I soon know they function according to a generally alien system of functioning that makes little match with my own. I know this because they are essentially multitrack and I am essentially mono. [...] [L]ike some animals, whatever I share in common with others, human or otherwise, what comes first for me is the recognition that I am in company of someone who has a basic sense of making sense of the world and themselves that is 'like mine.'" I keep asking myself—as I did when Matthew received the message "Donna says hi to Matthew": is this not a form of empathy, unaccounted for by most professional tests, statistics, and charts? Or should it be called by another name?

Writing these lines, it's hard for me not to think of my relationship with Matthew, based on so many misunderstandings, invalid projections, and false expectations from my side; and met on his by sheer incomprehension and a sense of dependency that angered him at times, but to which he grew more and more accustomed. He became friendlier, calling me by my first name more often than "Dad" (to which he remained ambivalent, while he never addressed me as "Father"). In his own way, and particularly when I was not present, he expressed affection toward me. When I was out of town, during the last years of his life, he even missed me. He would ask Uca: "When is Matei coming back? He is a better cook than you!" I enjoyed preparing for him tasty vegetarian meals, always from fresh produce, with just the right amount of olive oil and the spices that I knew he liked—transforming his palate into that of a rather sophisticated vegetarian gourmet; which doesn't mean that he minded eating canned vegetables or TV dinners; although he would prefer (tacitly, reluctantly when I was present) my cooking, voicing his praise only when I was away for longer periods of time. He must have been the first to realize that we belonged to different species, that real, profound communication between us (unlike his communication beyond words with Phil, his mentor, or with his long-time friend Julian, or even with his mother, who was infinitely more patient with him) was out of the question.

Things may have become a little more tolerable for him during the last decade of his life when, prompted by a reflective and self-reflective perusal of Asperger's paper, as I noted in my memoir, and by more recent readings, I became aware that I myself belonged to what is now called the "broader autism phenotype." Of course, this is a vague notion that could be applied to many people who function perfectly in society but tend to be somewhat withdrawn, less sociable—in the sense of gregarious—more introverted, more solitary by vocation, more distant in their relation with others. At any rate, I still belonged to a different species, perhaps not that far removed from his own, but different. And even small differences can lead to major incompatibilities.

As I said before, I want and need to learn as much as possible about autism—and if precise, certain knowledge is beyond reach, I want at least to keep up with new areas of research, new ways of questioning, new hypotheses, and new testimonies of parents, or of the few people with autism who can write and tell their story. Very recently I came across a book by Simon Baron-Cohen, *The Essential Difference: The Truth about the Male and Female Brain* (2003). I have mentioned him in my memoir with regard to his earlier volume, *Mindblindness: An Essay on Autism and Theory of Mind* (1995), and I have read other works by him and his collaborators. I would like to say a few words here about *The Essential Difference* and the thoughts it provoked in a layman like myself, although one with some direct parental experience of autism. But before I do so, I will offer a few purely subjective reactions to my readings on autism—this one included—over the last year or so, that is, after Matthew's death. I mention them here because they are germane to both my general acceptance of Baron-Cohen's thesis, that autism is probably a case of the "extreme male brain," and my criticism of its limitations (as I suggested earlier, certain forms of autistic empathy do exist and should not be glossed over). The reminiscences brought forth by my readings on autism are also relevant, I think, to the non-professional, and even anti-professional, views of people with autism and of parents of autistic children, of which I will speak later. I must confess: I cannot read anything about autism with detachment. How could I? My aim in this memoir has been to draw a portrait of Matthew, in order to understand him better. *Him*—and others like him—and myself in relationship to him.

For me, such reading is, on a personal level, also a way of reviving Matthew in my mind. I see him through the pages I peruse (however dry and theoretical they are), as if they were windows onto his past and mine at various ages: from infancy through his essentially happy preschool years, through elementary, middle, and high school, and after graduation, through the jobs Matthew held as a young man, and even—projecting, musing, surmising—through later stages of his life in a possible future he missed. For, however absurd this may seem, I continue to imagine his future as if he were alive. Even though some of the descriptions of autism I come across do not fit him, or do so only partially, his image asserts itself vividly through those very differences or contrasts. Reading has always been for me, however vicariously, an opportunity for self-reading. Matthew's image between the lines—the result of an unintended but unavoidable personal projection—often acquires an amazing precision, poignant and immaterial, that gradually dissolves into his broad, kind smile—which may have been, as some writers maintain, nothing more than a defense mechanism against the incomprehensible world of others, a delicate and inviting mask. But I cannot convince myself that there was no genuine sensitivity or goodness behind Matthew's magnetic smile—my fondest memory of him. On certain occasions his smile may indeed have been defensive, hiding a fear of what, for him, was perhaps threatening in unanticipated social situations. However, there were many occasions in which his smile expressed a wide range of positive sentiments—from a confident love of younger children to a state of wonder and elation when he smiled to himself on his way back home from work, unaware that he might be observed; to the ingratiating smiles with which he asked a favor ("Dad, could you drive me to Borders? Please, please!"), to those full of grateful exultation when his request was granted.

But let me return to the main focus of my attention as I read Baron-Cohen's *The Essential Difference*. From the first page, the author states clearly and succinctly the thesis of the book: "The female brain is predominantly hard-wired for empathy. The male brain is predominantly hard-wired for understanding and building systems." The demonstration that follows, based on research, observation, and psychological tests, some of them devised by the author and his collaborators, is, or sounds, convincing. (I am easily, too easily, convinced by all sorts of theories about autism, even when they diverge or contradict one another; for many years I have avoided psychoanalytical studies of autism, for fear they might convince me.)

I would agree with Baron-Cohen that autism is, among other things, an illustration of "The Extreme Male Brain" (pp. 133–154). My agreement derives from my own intuition and from the intuition of a great specialist, Dr. Hans Asperger, who synthesized his diagnostic observations on autistic children in his important 1944 thesis, which I mentioned in my memoir in a diary entry from 1993 (an entry that records my self-scrutiny: another instance of my tendency toward self-reading). Baron-Cohen refers to that work, too, quoting the following crucial passage: "The autistic personality is an extreme variant of male intelligence. Even within the normal variation, we find typical sex differences in intelligence."

Baron-Cohen then writes: "Autism spectrum conditions . . . appear to affect males far more than females. In people diagnosed with high-functioning autism or AS [Asperger's syndrome], the sex ratio is at least *ten males to every female* [emphasis in the original]. This too suggests that autism spectrum conditions are heritable. Interestingly, the sex ratio in autism spectrum conditions has not been investigated as much as perhaps it should have been, given that Nature has offered us a big clue about the cause of the condition" (p. 137). The superior Asperger types can sometimes marry and have children (but in those cases the wife, as Baron-Cohen points out, needs to be what he calls "a saint"), and have brilliant careers. A highly interesting case, described in the chapter "A Professor of Mathematics" (pp. 155—169) is that of Richard Borcherds, a professor at Cambridge University and a recipient of the Fields Medal, the highest distinction in mathematics, equivalent to a Nobel Prize in other disciplines. Interviewed by Baron-Cohen, Borcherds appears unaware of the huge gap in social understanding between himself and others. This cannot help reminding me of Matthew: "He was a master of mathematical judgment, but had hardly left first base in relation to social judgment. Social oddness is the first key symptom of AS. I asked him, for example, if he thought any of his behavior was socially odd or unusual. He said he couldn't think of anything in particular [. . .]. I asked him if there was anything else that he thought he did differently to others. 'No,' he said. What about communication, the second of the key symptoms of AS? Was there anything different about that? He could not think of anything, though he admitted he was not much of a conversationalist. From his perspective, talk was for finding out what you needed, and not much beyond that. I thought that he omitted to mention a function of language, which is to communicate your thoughts and feelings to another person, and to find out how they might be feeling or thinking. I said as much, but he said that was not really of interest to him" (p. 157).

Matthew, as I have pointed out, didn't feel that he was that different from others because, as he used to put it, "everybody is different." But he was not without interest in the feelings of others. When I complained: "I feel sick" or "I feel rotten," he showed concern and, in his awkward way, tried to console me. He was sensitive to pain—to the obvious signs of physical pain in others—and would exclaim "I am sorry, I am so sorry" when someone in his presence accidentally hurt himself. But more subtle variations in mood escaped him. The thoughts of others held no particular interest for him, but when he was in a really good mood and someone made some general statement, he seemed to enjoy playing with it, turning it upside down, even when he knew he was wrong: it was his naïve way of participating in the game of conversation, perhaps of being playful, the pleasure of a humorous reversal of the obvious, which he sometimes pursued at great length, giving all sorts of cockeyed reasons why he was right (but I need to stress: being conscious all along that he was wrong).

He rarely communicated his own feelings and states of mind when he was down; in the periods when he obscurely, unconsciously, organically sensed a coming seizure, he fell silent. Asked if he felt sick or had a headache (when he was eleven or twelve, for a year or so before his seizures started, he developed strong migraines that made him vomit and that worried us so much we took him to Children's Hospital in Cincinnati, only to be told that causes of migraine are mysterious), he covered his ears with his hands and invariably said "I am okay," but in an exasperated tone of voice that meant the contrary and also something like "Leave me alone!" He would sit for long periods with his elbows on the table, his head supported by his hands, eyes half-closed, refusing obstinately to complain. "I am okay, I am okay, I am okay, don't worry." He took everything as if it *had* to be the way it was. A year or so before his passing, when he had a stress fracture of a bone in his pelvis and had to lie down for over a month, moving around the house in a wheelchair, he never voiced the slightest complaint. He seemed satisfied if not happy to be the center of our attention, to learn how to use the wheelchair, to be obedient, to be an "ideal patient," as he had been at the National Institutes of Health several years back.

As for mathematics, I have noted in my memoir Matthew's strong attraction to numbers, to arithmetic operations and calculations, and to mathematical reasoning, in both elementary and middle school. He was proud of being good at math, of being praised by his teachers, of being placed in an advanced group, of being admired by his classmates. All this afforded him, at least in his own eyes, a certain status among his peers at school, allowing him to ignore their taunting and teasing, which went on even as they recognized his mathematical talent. In high school, however, he had a harder time keeping pace (he was helped by private tutors). The reason for this was, I think, the onset of epilepsy and the medication he was put on to control his seizures. This medication, in ever-increasing dosages, may have impaired his memory. According to one of his tutors in calculus, a very talented young mathematician working on his Ph.D., Matthew had a natural and quick understanding of what was being explained to him, he "saw" mathematical relations, but also quickly forgot what he had learned. At any rate, he thoroughly enjoyed doing math on a one-on-one basis with his tutor. For him it was like playing a game—he always eagerly awaited his tutor—but his game did not improve because of the frailty of his long-term memory.

This impairment may have led to Matthew's strange sense of time, reduced to a narrow present, to an uncertain, limited past, and hence to an equally uncertain, perhaps anxious, future, of which he preferred not to think. "I forget a lot," Matthew would readily admit. As for the future, when asked what he would like to be when he grew up, he was always puzzled, and responded with his easy-way-out to questions he did not understand: "I don't know," sometimes adding: "How would I know?" I wonder if memory is not, to a very large extent, responsible not only for our sense of the past, but also for our perception of the future, for our ability to make plans, to daydream (timidly, ambitiously), to form life projects, to see ourselves in wished-for situations. I remember how sad I was when I heard Matthew say: "I forget a lot" and then stressing, with exasperation: "I forget a lot—and so what?" And so what? And so what? This was one of Matthew's metaphysically most unanswerable questions: *And so what?*

Empathizing may be "modular," that is, independent from other mental processes, independent also from the systematizing ability of the extreme male brain, as Baron-Cohen suggests—which, in passing, would superficially confirm but ultimately ruin his whole argument. For modularity doesn't seem to explain why autistic people, while empathizing imperfectly or clumsily, if at all, with "normal" people, empathize fully and even passionately (admittedly a cold passion, but a passion nonetheless) with people like themselves. In the literature about autism I have read during the last year, this characteristic—of which Matthew's strong, obvious joy of being with other autistics made me aware—is mentioned in two books. To the first, *Autism: An Inside-Out Approach* by Donna Williams, I have already referred. The second is *Elijah's Cup,* by Valerie Paradiž (2002), a gripping and insight-provoking memoir by the mother of an autistic son.

For Donna Williams, the reciprocal recognition and empathy between persons with autism seems to derive from some kind of immediate intuition or even instinct. Using the term "system" entirely differently from Baron-Cohen and other professionals, she means by it simply a way of making sense of the world, from childhood on, in reaction to sensory stimuli (sounds—including tones of voice—colors, smells, sensations of touch and texture, tastes). There are two systems: "multi-track" in the case of "normal" individuals, and "single-track" in the case of autistic people. The latter can be easily overwhelmed by a variety of simultaneous impressions and thus produce a dramatic, paralyzing sensory overload. The autistic individual's sensory hypersensitivity is caused by their single-track or serial mode of processing stimuli and explains why there is such a gap between the autistic mind and the "normal" individual's capability of using a multi-track system of processing and patterning information so that it is socially acceptable. The key word here is "acceptability." There is no possibility of reading other minds, when the other minds tend to impose (however gently) their own interpretations, socially validated, on the mind of the autistic person.

As soon as I got a copy of Valerie Paradiž's memoir about her son Elijah, I read it straight through without putting it down, during an afternoon and a night of insomnia (which didn't diminish my attention) in late January 2004. I related easily to the author—an academic in the humanities like myself, although from a younger generation. The writers from whom she quotes—"high-brow" writers from Kafka to Gertrude Stein to Wittgenstein to Marjorie Perloff on Wittgenstein—are all quite familiar to me (actually, Marjorie Perloff, who published her book *Wittgenstein's Ladder* in 1996, is a close personal friend; the world is indeed a small place). I was fascinated with Elijah's development between the ages of two and ten, as well as with his mother's poignant but ultimately successful attempt to understand and identify her son's needs, within the emerging conception of autism as *not* a "mental disease" but as a "way of life," and even a "culture" with its own history, which she reconstructs in the course of her book. (She brings in vivid biographical details when speaking of famous personalities with autistic or Asperger-like features, such as Albert Einstein, the philosopher Ludwig Wittgenstein, or the pop artist Andy Warhol.)

In moral terms, Valerie Paradiž sets a wonderful parental example, and her book is an impressive testimony of what is involved in discovering, through love, the fragile, demanding, and beautiful otherness of one's "disabled" offspring. Of course, Elijah reminded me—by symmetrical contrast, analogy, as well as difference—of Matthew. His seizure disorder, unlike Matthew's, started early on, at age two, and fortunately he could be weaned off medication before entering school. In Matthew's case, the onset was at age thirteen and, after an interruption of nearly three years, the seizures came back with increasing intensity and frequency, uncontrollable by medication, leading to his premature death in one of the rare cases of "Sudden Unexplained Death in Epilepsy." (But how rare are such cases? Among the cards we received from members of our small community, who had read the obituary I wrote for the local paper, there were two which described absolutely similar recent deaths of young people with epilepsy.)

Among several other similarities, I was struck by Elijah's question to his mother, one day after coming home from school ("Am I crazy?"), which seemed to echo, over the years, Matthew's harrowing question to Uca in 1986, when he was nine and we were all three having breakfast: "Am I an idiotic person?" By then, he had developed his own method of blunting or ignoring stigmatizing language: the concept of "abnormality" had no place in his mind. Moreover, he never used such language himself. Derision, mocking, insulting, verbally injuring others were absent from his own sensibility; he had a clear feeling of justice and fair play. When others mocked him—which, as he grew up, became extremely rare—he preferred not to respond in kind.

Uca and I were certainly aware of the autistic empowerment movement, started under the umbrella of Autism Society of America (ASA) by Jim Sinclair and others—a movement that grew increasingly independent from the more traditional-professional oriented ASA—but we didn't follow it, as perhaps we should have, due to Matthew's more and more acute seizure disorder, which made him unfit to go to the Autreat summer camp (a retreat for autistic people organized by Jim Sinclair and Autism Network International, or ANI). Valerie Paradiž's account of her and Elijah's participation in Autreat is one of the most interesting parts of her book. The whole idea of ANI, I think, is based on the intriguing empathy among autistic people. As Valerie Paradiž puts it: "Although the core organizers of ANI are all 'high-functioning,' the group extends its vision of independence and autistic self-awareness to the entire spectrum."

In this respect, I feel, professional research is lagging. How can autistic people read the minds of other autistic people? The explanation seems simple but the consequences of taking stock of this fundamental fact could revolutionize the whole theory-of-mind psychology as it is now established. For one thing, it could make it more sensitive to cultural differences and broader anthropological questions. At any rate, the notion of a culture of autism and of a sort of "normality" within that culture—including the possibility of spontaneous empathy—merits a more systematic exploration.

That autism is a disability—and a tragic one, at that—is undeniable. But it is the responsibility of our society, insofar as it wishes to be considered humane, to understand this disability as it seems to understand blindness or deafness. As Valerie Paradiž writes about Jim Sinclair: "Clearly, he was [. . .] an intellectual descendant of Helen Keller and Louis Braille. And like these early activists, who transformed the paradigm for the deaf and blind, Jim's pioneering ideas on autism were being received with ambivalence, and sometimes outright rejection, by major organizations like the Autism Society of America (ASA) and More Advanced Autistic People (MAAP). [. . .] Jim was one of a handful of autistics at the time who were introducing basic concepts of self-advocacy. He modeled his ideas on the successes of the deaf community and other groups within the disability movement" (p. 137). About attempts to "normalize" autistic behavior, Sinclair observes with common sense: "Expecting that we act 'normal' socially is sort of like expecting blind people to drive cars instead of teaching them skills to use public transportation."

A measure of the (partial) success of this movement was, at least insofar as Matthew was concerned, the creation of the group ABLE in Bloomington. At its monthly meetings for supper in various restaurants, and occasionally for attending basketball games, in Indianapolis or here in our university town with a fine basketball team, Matthew participated with great pleasure. The real problem for autistics is how to deal, most of the time, with solitude. As a matter of fact, social interaction for people with autism (even if they interact happily with other autistics in summer camps such as Autreat) remains a marginal part of their day-to-day life, in which they are surrounded and protected by "normal" people, with whom they communicate only superficially or not at all. Who will teach them how to deal—if they are not mathematical geniuses, or logical geniuses like Wittgenstein—with solitude?

That was, I think, Matthew's greatest problem, compounded by his lack of long-term memory and therefore by his reduced power of anticipation. He spent an inordinate amount of time playing video games such as Nintendo or watching TV—mostly Disney or programs on Nickelodeon, but also the pseudo-violence of professional wrestling shows, in which, I would guess, he appreciated more the well-rehearsed loud faking than the apparent violence; and of course sports, about which he knew a lot, and which offered him a means of broader social interaction. But his was an essentially solitary mind. I see it as a pure mental sky, transparently blue as some late summer skies, not crossed by cloudy reveries, nostalgias, memories, projects, or even hopes. In a way his forgetfulness was a blessing for him, because he did not recall his seizures and their aftermath, and so he could fully enjoy his moments of happiness, which came to him as gifts out of the blue, all the more exciting as they were rarely if ever expected.

What continues to amaze me is that Matthew had, naturally, such a good—and perhaps I should stress, *beautiful* and *lovable*—character. We failed to teach him how to pretend to be "normal." He was who he was. He may have become momentarily angry when he was misunderstood by his parents. As for the others' misunderstandings, after his early years in grade school, when he responded as a bully to taunting, he tended to be amused by them later on or to simply ignore them. He was gentle and tolerant. His essential, untaught, spontaneous, luminous goodness remained the same. And when he smiles, as I remember him, he smiles not only with his lips or his eyes or his face, but with his entire being.

BLOOMINGTON, FEBRUARY 2004

Works Cited

Asperger, Hans. "'Autistic Psychopathy' in Childhood." In *Autism and Asperger Syndrome,* ed. Uta Frith, 37–92. Cambridge: Cambridge University Press, 1991.

Ayres, Jean A. *Sensory Integration and the Child.* Los Angeles: Western Psychological Services, 1979.

Baron-Cohen, Simon. *Mindblindness: An Essay on Autism and Theory of Mind.* Cambridge, Mass.: MIT Press, 1995.

———. *The Essential Difference: The Truth about the Male and the Female Brain.* New York: Basic Books, 2003.

Bateson, Gregory, ed. *Steps to an Ecology of Mind.* New York: Ballantine Books, 1972.

Bettelheim, Bruno. *The Empty Fortress: Infantile Autism and the Birth of the Self.* New York: Free Press, 1967.

Caillois, Roger. *Man, Play, and Games.* New York: Schocken Books, 1979.

Calinescu, Matei. *Rereading.* New Haven, Conn.: Yale University Press, 1993.

Diagnostic and Statistical Manual of Mental Disorders: DSM-III-R. 3rd ed., rev. Washington, D.C.: American Psychiatric Association, 1987.

Frith, Uta, ed. *Autism and Asperger Syndrome.* Cambridge: Cambridge University Press, 1991.

———. *Autism: Explaining the Enigma*. Oxford and Cambridge, Mass.: Basil Blackwell, 1989.

Grandin, Temple. *Emergence: Labeled Autistic*. Novato, Calif.: Arena Press, 1986.

———. *Thinking in Pictures: And Other Reports from my Life with Autism*. Foreword by Oliver Sacks. New York: Doubleday, 1995.

Huizinga, Johan. *Homo Ludens: A Study of the Play-Element in Culture*. Boston: Beacon Press, 1962.

Journal of Autism and Developmental Disorders. New York: Plenum Press.

Kanner, Leo. *Childhood Psychosis: Initial Studies and New Insights*. Washington, D.C.: V. H. Winston, 1973.

Paradiž, Valerie. *Elijah's Cup: A Family's Journey into the Community and Culture of High-Functioning Autism and Asperger's Syndrome*. New York: Free Press, 2002.

Park, Clara Claiborne. *The Siege: The First Eight Years of an Autistic Child*. Boston: Little, Brown & Co., 1982.

Piaget, Jean. *The Language and Thought of the Child*. New York: Meridian Books, 1955.

Picard, Michel. *La lecture comme jeu*. Paris: Editions de Minuit, 1986.

Sacks, Oliver. *An Anthropologist on Mars*. New York: Knopf, 1995.

Tinbergen, Niko, and Elisabeth A. Tinbergen. *Autistic Children: New Hope for a Cure*. London and Boston: Allen & Unwin, 1983.

Wellman, Henry M. *The Child's Theory of Mind*. Cambridge, Mass.: MIT Press, 1990.

Whiten, Andrew, ed. *Natural Theories of Mind: Evolution, Development, and Simulation in Everyday Mindreading*. Oxford and Cambridge, Mass.: Basil Blackwell, 1991.

Williams, Donna. *Autism: An Inside-Out Approach*. London and Bristol, Pa.: Jessica Kingsley Publishers, 1996.

———. *Nobody Nowhere: The Extraordinary Autobiography of an Autistic*. New York: Times Books, 1992.

Wing, Lorna, ed. *Early Childhood Autism: Clinical, Educational, and Social Aspects*. Oxford and New York: Pergamon Press, 1976.

MATEI CALINESCU is Professor Emeritus of Comparative Literature at Indiana University, Bloomington, where he has taught since immigrating to the United States from Communist Romania in 1973. His books in English include *Five Faces of Modernity: Modernism, Avant-Garde, Decadence, Kitsch, Postmodernism* (1987) and *Rereading* (1993).